pilates

a beginner's guide

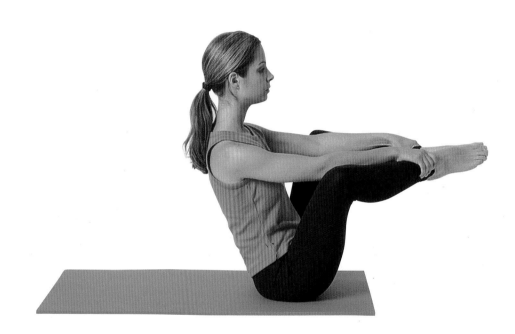

pilates
a beginner's guide

Roger Brignell

D&S
BOOKS

First published in 2001 by D&S Books

© 2001 D&S Books

D&S Books
Cottage Meadow, Bocombe,
Parkham, Bideford
Devon, England
EX39 5PH

e-mail us at:-
enquiries.dspublishing@care4free.net

This edition printed 2001

ISBN 1-903327-23-7

Editorial Director: Sarah King
Editor: Sarah Harris
Project Editor: Yvonne Worth
Designer: Dave Jones
Photography: Paul Forrester/Colin Bowling

Distributed in the UK & Ireland by
Bookmart Limited
Desford Road
Enderby
Leicester LE9 5AD

Distributed in Australia by
Herron Books
39 Commercial Road
Fortitude Valley
Queensland 4006

1 3 5 7 9 10 8 6 4 2

Contents

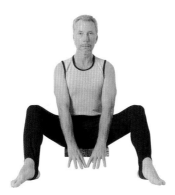

Introduction

Pilates is a multi-muscle exercise technique which has at its heart two fundamental beliefs:

1 That exercise which does not involve the brain is wasted.

2 That a strong central core – which requires development of the muscles in order to support and stabilise the spine – is a prerequisite for attaining a strong and healthy body.

The exercises as prescribed and described originally are functional. It is the exerciser's own bodyweight that provides the training resistance and as such educates the muscles to support the body efficiently and effectively at all times. The rationale for this is that this is precisely what the body is designed to do.

The Pilates method takes as its starting point the adjustment of posture to make the individual feel taller and look trimmer. Practicing the exercises does not build big muscles but does increase strength where it is needed. It also stretches and lengthens any muscles that have become too short and tight. The natural result is increased flexibility and joint mobility.

There are no age or fitness barriers to participation and even those with injuries can, subject to the agreement of their medical advisers, participate and – more importantly – benefit from the Pilates technique.

The emphasis of Pilates is on the development of a mind and body that are healthy because they work together, and through this working together the focus is on achieving a healthier life.

As people have become less convinced about the efficacy of traditionally based exercise programmes, a more holistic, mind-body approach is increasingly finding favour. Traditional programmes tend to focus on isolating individual muscles and trying to work them separately from the rest of the body in order to achieve fitness, but they do not necessarily improve general health – nor is that their aim.

Clearly in an era that has begun to focus on the mind-body movement as the way forwards for individuals seeking to stay fit and healthy, the Pilates method has an immediate and obvious appeal. This, coupled with the fact that for many years the method has been practiced and taught by professional dancers, many of whom have subsequently become involved in the fitness industry as class instructors, demonstrates why the method has grown so much in popularity over the past few years. A case of the being the right system in the right place at the right time.

Whilst there is no doubt an element of fashion in its current popularity, it is undeniably effective in achieving results. This is why it has been taught and practiced for more than ninety years and why people are still becoming 'Pilates converts' today.

WHO WAS JOSEPH PILATES?

Joseph Hubertus Pilates was born in (or near) Dusseldorf in Germany in 1880 and died in New York in 1967. Since he dedicated the greater part of his life to promoting the idea of a healthy and fit body and mind, he would doubtless have felt that living to a great age was testament to the effectiveness of his exercise programmes.

Joseph Pilates was a very sickly child. He suffered from rickets, from rheumatic fever and from what is now often thought of as a very modern disease – asthma. As a result he was determined to make himself as fit and as strong and healthy as he could. While still young he studied and exercised and eventually became a competent skier, diver and gymnast. He took up bodybuilding and succeeded sufficiently well to be invited to pose for anatomical charts in adolescence. His range of sources for his personal exercise regime included yoga, self-defence and dance as well as weight training. He also spent some time training as a circus acrobat.

Introduction

No doubt feeling that he had discovered a secret worth communicating, he took his training method to the outside world and by 1914 was teaching self-defence to detectives in London. At the beginning of World War I, still in London, he was interned because of his nationality. Unperturbed, he decided that his fellow internees on the Isle of Man were in need of help to improve their fitness and keep them healthy and he instructed them accordingly. It was later claimed that the fact that not one of these internees died in the influenza epidemic was a direct result of his fitness training.

Also at this time he began adding springs as part of the resistance training machines that were being used to help in the rehabilitation programmes for amputees in the camp hospitals. One can see here perhaps the beginnings of the equipment-based exercises that he later developed into his programmes. After the war he went back to Germany – this time as a trainer for the police force.

Eventually he decided to emigrate to the United States and in 1926 he and his wife set up a fitness studio at 939 Eighth Avenue, New York. The studio and the method became popular with ballet dancers such as George Balanchine and Martha Graham and soon gymnasts, sportspeople and actors, drawn particularly by the successes his methods achieved for those with injuries, began to frequent the studio.

WHY HAS THE PILATES METHOD TAKEN SO LONG TO GET KNOWN?

Joseph Pilates wrote only a couple of books during his lifetime. They concerned themselves with advanced forms of his exercises and with what today may seem overly complex first drafts of the 'Pilates Philosophy'. The reason that he concentrated solely on the advanced forms of his exercises is not difficult to understand. The clientele at the studio were, in general, fit individuals. As far as Pilates was concerned, his readership was going to comprise of people, like his clients, who had already achieved a reasonable level of fitness. He was certainly not writing for beginners.

It is easy to see that this high-mindedness would have had the effect of making the exercise programme seem not only physically difficult but in some ways inappropriate and inaccessible to the average individual. It was not until the fitness boom of the 1970s and the advent of mass aerobic classes that the Pilates technique began to seep into the wider consciousness. Indeed, many classes were both designed and taught by people who had had previous dance training and who, as a result, had come into contact with the Pilates exercises and allowed this to influence their teaching in fitness classes.

Even then the popular fitness movement placed a strong emphasis on cardiovascular exercise and fat burning rather than focusing on what the muscles of the body are actually designed for and how to make them fit for what is required of them in today's world. This latter issue has only begun to be a readily accepted in the past five years or so and it is this above all else that has been the major influence in the spectacular growth in interest in Pilates exercises.

Introduction

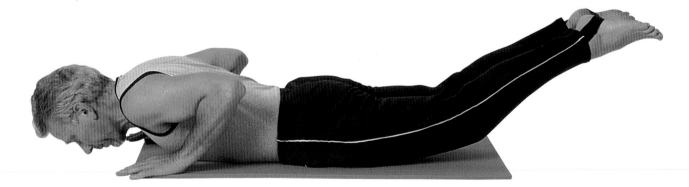

The current emphasis on functional exercise – that is to say exercise which supports and enhances the function of muscles and joints as they are used by the individual in his or her everyday life – has been very much led by the results of academic research. What has emerged from this kind of research (and what is still emerging) is that that a strong 'core' is an absolute pre-requisite for all physical activity.

Thus exercise practitioners looked around for ready-made programmes that laid emphasis on this notion of strengthening the 'core' and Pilates was ready and waiting.

THE PILATES' ATTITUDE TO LIFE

Given Joseph Pilates' early life experience it is not at all surprising that at the heart of his approach to living lies the idea that in order to live a healthy and happy life you need a body that will never let you down – and most of us would agree with him heartily.

Pilates did, however, take the whole thing further. He argued that the flexibility and fluidity of childhood movement is something that we have no reason to lose as we grow older. The only thing that makes us less flexible and more tentative in adulthood is an accumulation of inappropriate postural and movement habits. Pilates believed that if we are serious about our health we can lose these habits (or at least the majority of them) by taking control. By this he meant making our muscles behave in a way that we consciously decide upon, rather than in a way that has been developed by careless habit and neglect.

Here Pilates' views are very much in tune with modern ways of thinking. He believed that we must each take responsibility for our own health and that we must develop an attitude of strength and confidence in relation to our bodies so that we can be in charge. This is another reason why the Pilates technique is so popular at the moment – the philosophy does seem to be in line with the thinking of our time.

In some ways this makes embarking on a Pilates course easier since the values of self-reliance and self-help are very much ones to which we adhere these days. What we all need to be sure about though is that we keep these ideas conscious, rather than unconscious, in our exercise sessions so that the determination to be in control of our bodies is at the front of our minds while we perform the programme.

Principles of Pilates

Your first contact with the Pilates exercise programme may make you feel that it is just an eclectic fusion of a number of other approaches. You may recognise elements of yoga, movements reminiscent of Alexander Technique, dance movements, everyday exercises from the gym as well as childhood gymnastics.

This is true to a certain extent since this is how Joseph Pilates studied to develop a fitness regime for himself. As he found elements in other programmes (and other philosophies) that worked for him as he was trying to overcome his childhood weaknesses, he both adopted and adapted them initially for himself and then later for his clients and pupils. He took on board the elements that he found to work the best and discarded anything that did not pass the tests of practicality.

What makes the approach unique is Pilates' insistence on a number of 'principles'. These too may in some ways sound familiar but what makes them important is the fact that they come as a package – no part is optional if the Pilates exercise programme is to work effectively. The eight 'principles' are an inherent part of the effort that is required.

These principles are:

- Concentration
- Control
- Centre
- Breath
- Fluidity
- Precision
- Routine
- Isolation

It is not always easy to explain all the principles in words but as they are such an important and integral part of the method we need to spend some time reviewing their meanings here.

CONCENTRATION

This principle lies at the very heart of the Pilates method. Pilates is not an exercise programme that allows you to switch off your mind and let your body run on automatic. The mind must be alert at all times, controlling every movement. Concentration is what connects mind and body and allows you to block out everything but the movement you are trying to achieve.

Without concentration the Pilates method cannot exist. Many of the movements appear to be deceptively simple. Concentration allows you to focus both on those muscles performing the movement and those facilitating the movement by stabilising the parts of your body which are required to remain immobile.

In practical terms this means that when you are performing your routine you need to be sure that you are as relaxed as you can be, in surroundings that are as free of distraction as possible, and with enough privacy to provide the certainty that you will not be interrupted.

CONTROL

The idea behind control in the Pilates method is much like the ideas in yoga or even in weight training. For the exercising muscle to work effectively it must do exactly what it is asked to do – no more and no less. Additionally control is vital in order to ensure that injuries do not occur. In many ways this can be one of the more problematic principles to incorporate into your routine. What you will be trying to achieve is a smooth and relaxed set of movements but these can only be attained as a result of both concentration and of minute control of the relevant muscle movements.

When you first start the programme, imagining (visualising) the relevant muscles working may be of great assistance. You will almost certainly not get it exactly right first time – it takes practice. Remember that babies take time to learn to walk – and they have no distractions and no time pressures. Making mistakes is part of our condition. It's one of the ways we learn things.

Principles of Pilates

Pilates called what we refer to as the centre – 'the powerhouse'. By this he meant that when a body is functioning correctly in terms of its muscular activity the source of all the power and movement is located at the centre of the body. At this centre (the point approximately two inches below the navel) we have a large number of muscles – the muscles of the abdomen and the lumbar spine, as well as those of the hips and buttocks. These muscles, as is normally the case in nature, have more than one function. At the most obvious level they support and protect the soft organs of the abdomen. As we begin to understand more and more about the structure and the biomechanics of our bodies this function appears increasingly to be secondary to the function of supporting and protecting the lumbar spine. This area is sometimes now called the central core and current thinking suggests that without a strong central core most forms of exercise – and even ordinary everyday activities – will inevitably result in injury.

Originally humans were not designed to stand erect, and the only reason we can do is due to our central core. It is not surprising, therefore, that when viewed in this particular context we need to keep the centre strong.

Pilates was preaching this particular principle more than 50 years ago. As far as he was concerned, energy and control for all the exercises begin in the core and flow out to the extremities. This is a total contrast to more traditional forms of exercise in which the limbs are the primary focus for the initiation of muscular activity. Centring allows lengthening and stretching to take place without the risk of injury to the spine. Here the muscles of the core can been viewed as the conductors of a muscle orchestra. They keep time and control the rhythm and strength of the movements of the other muscles.

BREATH

Breathing and breath control are at the heart of the Pilates exercises. As a teacher I have found that this is one of the hardest aspects of the technique for students to master. The principle is relatively easy to learn but the application itself is more difficult. Pilates was once again ahead of scientific knowledge in his emphasis not only on the correct rhythm for the breath but – more importantly in some ways – in his insistence on the correct technique. His concern was that whilst exercising most people tend to either breathe with just the upper part of the chest or to hold their breath during certain phases of the exercise. At best this will inhibit the precision of the movements and in many instances it makes it impossible to complete the movement accurately.

In modern life we have a tendency to use the chest to control our breath, i.e. to breathe deeply we tend to use the muscles between our ribs to lift the ribcage, which results in a flow of air into the top part of the lungs but does not supply new air to the lower lungs at all. Clearly in terms of supplying oxygen (which is absorbed through the walls of the lung) to the working muscles this is very inefficient since something less than one third of the lung's surface will have new oxygen to distribute.

Principles of Pilates

If we could breathe in such a way as to fill the whole lung with new air the efficiency of our oxygen supply could be increased enormously. And we have been supplied with a mechanism for doing just this. It is called lateral breathing and in some ways it resembles the kind of breathing that singers and actors are taught and which for them involves the use of the diaphragm. For our purposes it is sufficient to focus on the lower part of the rib cage and the muscles of the abdomen. Using these muscles to control breathing results in an expansion of the lungs outwards (laterally) rather than lifting upwards and this means that new air is brought right to the bottom of the lungs. This results in increased efficiency.

The next step is then to co-ordinate the breath with the exercise, in order to establish the rhythm. Although each exercise has its own rhythm, the general principle is that as you prepare for the movement you breathe in; as you perform it (Effort) you breathe out (Exhale) and as you recover to repeat the movement you breathe in again.

FLUIDITY

Fluidity is not the exact word that Pilates used to describe this aspect of his exercise programme. He, and others, talked about flowing movements – the idea is that repetitions of the individual exercises, and the sequence of exercises, are designed to be performed as a whole. Each individual exercise should be performed as a continuous movement, with no 'rests' between repetitions, and the change to the next exercise in the sequence should be, as near as possible, a seamless meld. There should be

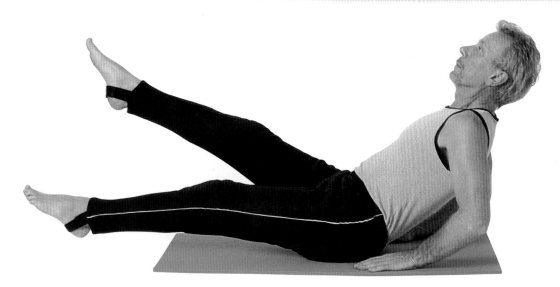

no variation in speed between exercises and the range of movement in each should be the same, so that the sequence viewed as a whole resembles the movement of a metronome.

In my view this is a concept that relates more to how each individual 'feels' whilst performing the exercises rather than to how it looks. Only the performer can know whether it is right or wrong. This is because the timing mechanism that makes the exercises feel fluid, with a single rhythm that governs the whole, relates to the individual's own muscles and how they function.

PRECISION

Exactness in execution is the hallmark of the Pilates exercises. It is not an optional extra but central to the effectiveness of the whole process. When you are new to the sequences it can be hard to take into account all the instructions, to think about and control all the muscles that are being used and, at the same time, to move with precision. It is, however, essential, and time and effort spent in attaining precision at an early stage will be more than repaid in terms of the benefit that the exercises will bring. Without this precision the value of the routine is compromised, while with practice and patience precision becomes a beneficial habit.

Acquiring precision is undoubtedly difficult – gymnasts and acrobats spend the bulk of their professional lives endeavouring to do precisely this. In practical terms this will take a lot of time and concentration. It will

Principles of Pilates

also require you to develop the ability to visualise exactly how you are moving during each individual exercise. Using a large mirror while you are practicing can be very useful.

ROUTINE

This principle is similar to the idea of rehearsing for a theatrical performance or of repetition in terms of most exercise or dance routines. What it provides is familiarity and recognition with regard to the exercises. By establishing the routines (as long as we bring focus and concentration to the routine) we improve the way we execute the exercises and enhance the skills that we bring to the process.

ISOLATION

This principle seems to be the most misunderstood. What I believe Pilates intended to promote with his isolation principle is the idea that while you are focused and concentrating on a whole movement, the movement actually consists of isolated muscles or muscle groups co-operating in a precise and controlled fashion to produce the whole. Each of us is individual and unique with muscles, bones and joints that have spent (for most of us) years getting us into our unique shape. Attaining the necessary skills for this new exercise programme, in order to achieve the balanced body that the Pilates technique will build, requires different degrees of effort and different ways of isolating from each of us.

All of this may sound rather daunting. It may appear more like a commitment to a way of life rather than a simple exercise programme. Don't worry! It is surprisingly simple once a few of the basics have been mastered, so do not be put off by the descriptions above.

The principles of Pilates are, in my view, simply an organised statement of what is required to perform any exercise programme effectively.

Any athlete, gymnast, tennis or football player would lay claim to the principles of control, of focus (concentration), fluidity, precision, routine and isolation to effect integration. Breath and centring might be less obvious but weightlifters, swimmers and yoga practitioners would subscribe to the concepts even if they use them and think about them in slightly different terms. As a newcomer to Pilates these should be seen as a helpful set of clues rather than as a rigid set of rules.

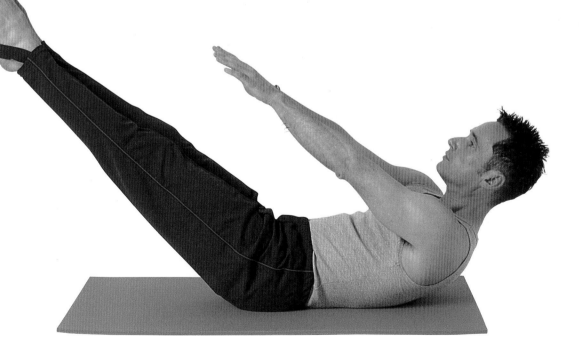

Who will benefit from Pilates?

Having made an attempt to explain what the Pilates method involves and to describe its underlying principles, who, then, should participate in the exercises and for whom are they suitable?

The answer is simple – just about anybody and everybody. Age is no barrier – I know people who have taken up a beginner's programme in their seventies. Nor is youth a bar, as the exercises are ideal for the developing bodies of the adolescent, far more so than many gym-based programmes. This is because there is no stress on growing bones, nor is excessive force applied to joints, ligaments and tendons that are not yet in tune with the newly acquired size and strength which adolescents enjoy. Provided that they are well advised and properly controlled and monitored those with back problems can participate and – more importantly – can benefit greatly from the exercises, as can those with joint problems. Many of the ordinary aches and pains that result from the strains of everyday life and poor posture the majority of us adopt in order to perform many of our tasks, can be alleviated by a well-constructed and rigorously performed Pilates programme.

Anyone who genuinely desires to have a longer, leaner look, improved posture and the sense of well being that comes from having muscles that do as they ought and a body that is under control should give Pilates a try.

You do not need to be fit before you start. You do not need to be an expert. All that is required is a level of commitment. In return you will get stronger, become more flexible and your silhouette will become longer and leaner. You will improve your posture, suffer from fewer aches and pains and have a lot more energy.

In addition you will make small, but noticeable, improvements to your respiratory efficiency and to your circulation. Your improved posture should reduce any headaches and back pain, your legs and arms will have improved muscle tone, your lymphatic drainage system will be improved and your immune system boosted. Finally, by developing core stability your stomach will be flatter and your abdominal muscles tighter. Extra benefits for those who participate in active pastimes come in the shape of fewer and less severe injuries.

Pilates will not by itself help you to lose weight, nor will it make your heart and lungs fit. For both of these you will need to make additional arrangements. (Some provision for cardio-respiratory exercise such as aerobics classes or walking/running three times a week is definitely advisable in terms of ensuring long-term health, provided that your doctor has no objections.)

I mention the importance of cardio-respiratory exercise at this point because there is currently a tendency to credit exercise as a cure-all. For muscles and for the skeleton the exercises described in this book are very potent for engendering functional well-being. By this I mean that the exercises make muscles, joints and bones strong for everyday living. The breathing technique also brings significant respiratory benefits, but Pilates exercises do not ask the heart to work very much harder than usual. For the heart to improve in function and for further development of the respiratory system some fairly hard (for the individual) physical exercise is desirable. Exercise that raises the heart rate and the respiratory rate significantly, for at least 20 minutes, no fewer than 3 times per week has a significant effect on health according to current U.K. medical recommendations.

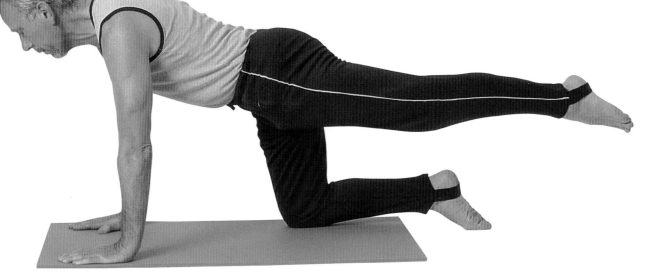

Preparation

 If you have come this far and have decided you want to continue, what do you need to do by way of preparation and how do you begin? It will be clear from what you have already read that the main requirement of the Pilates method is commitment.

There are also some concepts and some basic actions that need to be mastered before undertaking the programme. It is well worth learning these thoroughly before moving on, as they are employed in the execution of the majority of the exercises and are crucial to both the safe performance of the exercises and to maximising the beneficial effects.

I have already mentioned the concept of core stability more than once and this modern phrase accurately describes a concept that Pilates invented and which he called the 'powerhouse'. The 'powerhouse' comprises the various muscle groups found in the abdomen, lower back, buttocks and hips.

What is important about this core is that it not only controls accurate and precise movement but it is also the major component of effective and healthy posture. From here all Pilates movements are generated and therefore in order to perform any Pilates exercise it is important to know how to engage the powerhouse.

First, let me say that every one of us develops their own way of doing this as they practice, but to get started there are a number of tricks that can help. Perhaps most useful is the mechanism that we can all use to adjust our posture:

Most of us do not stand or sit well. The tendency is to allow our weight to sink into the core and for the core to accept the burden passively.

In contrast, healthy posture requires that the core actively supports the weight in these positions. This results in the removal of pressure from the back and a realignment of the spine, pelvis and hips to distribute the stress that results from our upright carriage more effectively.

Try to practice this in front of the mirror to start with. It will very soon become second nature.

Here is how healthy posture is achieved in the standing position.

- Place your feet at hip-width apart and parallel to each other.

- Soften your knees so that they are straight but not over-extended. You are aiming to have your weight evenly balanced between the front and back of each foot and evenly balanced between your feet. (As you do this you will feel your hips and spine move slightly more in line with each other and your weight will be directed vertically through your knee and hip joints).

- Focus now on the abdomen and pull up hard on the pelvic floor muscle (the one you use to interrupt urine flow) and at the same time pull in hard on your navel, pulling it towards the spine (this flattens your stomach and alters the curve in your lower back – you will feel weight lift up from this area of your back as you perform this action)

- Now go back to your feet and imagine that each foot is a rectangle. Ensure that your weight is now evenly distributed between each foot and between the four corners of each imaginary rectangle.

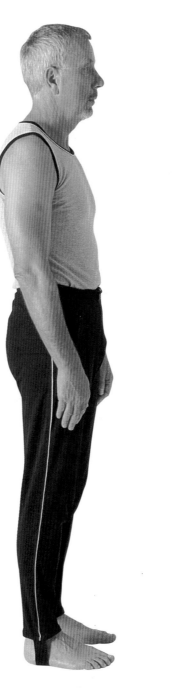

Here the spine is incorrect.

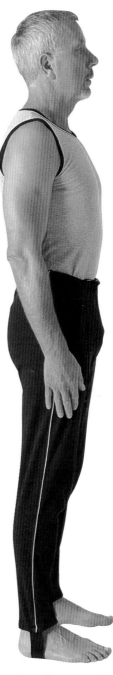

Standing correctly.

Preparation

- Focus on your head. Imagine there is a thread that runs up through your spine, through your neck and continues through the top of your skull vertically to the ceiling. Imagine that only the tension in the string keeps your body stretched upwards and your face looking straight ahead.
- Finally focus on your shoulders. Keep them relaxed and think about your shoulder blades. Try to keep them as far from each other as possible, arms hanging relaxed.

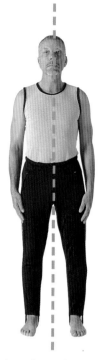

Imagine a thread running through your spine and up to the ceiling keeping your posture correct.

This may feel a little odd to start with but you will very soon get used to it. Practice it whenever you can – at the bus stop, doing the washing up, while cleaning your teeth. You will be surprised at how soon it becomes natural. And how quickly it starts to improve your silhouette.

What you will have noticed in the above description is that there are a lot of phrases asking you to imagine things happening. This is a technique that in modern times has been developed through sports sciences. Each and every one of us has been using such techniques since childhood, and although the origins probably date back to prehistory, sports and exercise psychologists have, more recently, discovered that visualisation is a very powerful tool when applied to the learning of new motor (muscle) skills. They have also found that it significantly reduces the time taken to acquire such skills.

At its very simplest the technique requires you to visualise whatever it is that you are trying to achieve, and to try to imagine what it feels like, the emotions that it makes you feel and so on. It also provides a way for talking about activities and parts of the body with which a lot of people will be unfamiliar and a way of recalling, with some precision, any new skill once it has been successfully performed.

Pilates teachers use it a lot as a method for describing how to achieve some of the basic moves in the repertoire because the moves by themselves are often somewhat unusual. As a result they can be difficult to imagine without some assistance. If you find that having mastered a certain move or exercise you prefer to visualise it using different imagery, this is very good. The ideas here are suggestions only, and should be taken as just that.

Along with visualisation, another technique to help you find and utilise the right muscles is very simply to touch the muscle that you are trying to use. This has the function of sending a message to the appropriate area of the brain, establishing a route as it were, for the reciprocal message back from the brain when it is required. If you do this two or three times for muscles that you have difficulty in activating, you will be surprised at the difference it makes when you need the muscle to work for you.

A healthy sitting posture is achieved in much the same way.

- Sit square in the chair with your feet parallel and flat on the floor, a hip width apart. The angle at the knee should be approximately 90°.
- Make sure that there is still some 'weight' in your feet. This way you will know that you are not leaning back too far.
- Exactly as for standing, pull up on your pelvic floor muscle and use the muscles of your lower abdomen to pull your navel as close to the spine as you are able. (You will feel the curve in your lower back change and tension in this area reduce).
- Lengthen your neck towards the ceiling (remember the thread through your spine and skull).
- Relax your shoulders and arms and place your shoulder blades as far apart as you can.

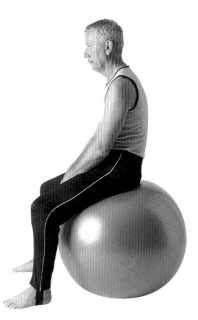

This shows an incorrect sitting position.

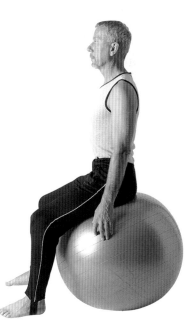

Here the sitting position is correct.

Preparation

Again when you first do this you may feel odd or uncomfortable. Don't be put off by this but persist. Usually within two weeks it will start to feel quite natural.

Much of the exercise programme we are going to perform is performed lying on our backs. Lying in the correct posture is important to achieving both safe and efficient execution of the exercises.

Lying correctly is simply an adaptation of the standing and sitting positions that we have talked about earlier.

- Lie on your back on the mat. Bend your knees, bringing your feet towards your buttocks. Your feet should be flat on the floor, about a hip-width apart and parallel to each other, and your arms relaxed and by your sides.
- Shoulders should be relaxed and pulled down. Try to keep your body long. This means lengthening your neck in just the same way as for sitting and standing.
- If your neck is not comfortable like this, a firm cushion or a folded towel underneath your head should make this better. In my experience the folded towel is useful for most people to start with and this can be dropped later.

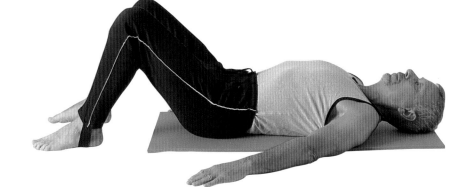

Correct posture for lying on your back.

This position is perfect for practising the basic control of the abdominal muscles that is required for most of the exercises and which will again very soon become second nature as you progress.

This abdominal control is very important and many teachers have used different ways to try to describe it.

As you are lying on the floor in the position described above, what is often called the hollow of your back will leave a gap between your spine and the mat. This is natural and desirable and the size of the gap will vary

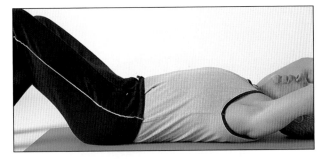

Round your spine so that you push
it in to the mat. Note how it feels.

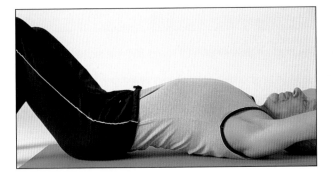

Now round your spine the other way so that it is curved as
far away as possible from the mat. Note how it feels.

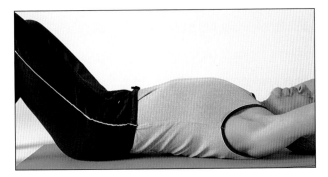

Next move your spine to a position that is
approximately half way between the two extremes.

from person to person. What most of us have become accustomed to however is to allow our abdominal muscles to relax completely when we lie down and this exaggerates this natural curvature of our spines. Here is the point at which it is important to introduce the concept of 'neutral spine'.

Once you have adopted the proper positions in the posture exercises (both seated and standing), you will find that if you take one hand and place it in the small of your back there is a curve. As I have said earlier all of us have such a curve to a greater or lesser extent, and for the sake of simplicity here I will call this curve 'neutral spine'.

When lying on the floor we need to re-establish this curve. To do this, lie on the mat as before, feet drawn in towards the buttocks, flat on the floor and about hip width apart. Repeat the whole process two or three times until you are happy that you have found 'half way'. This is 'neutral spine.'

The reason why this concept and this position is important is that a lot of the exercises require you to be able to hold the spine in this position, using your lower abdominal muscles, whilst performing movements with the limbs and or thorax (chest). It is here that the concept of the 'core' becomes a practical reality.

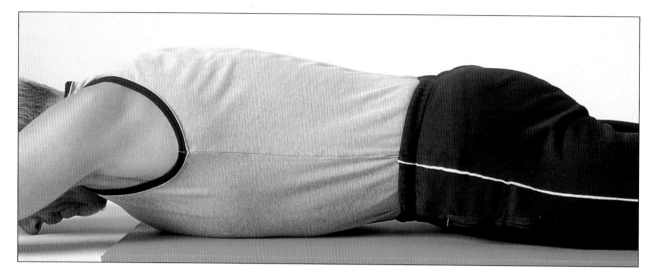

Activating the lower abdominal muscles – those muscles that will allow you to maintain the position of your spine in neutral while you are challenged to move your legs and arms – is not always easy. We described the process whilst illustrating good posture. Focus now on the abdomen and pull up hard on your pelvic floor muscle. At the same time pull in hard on your navel, pulling it towards your spine. This flattens your stomach and alters the curve in your lower back. You will feel weight lift up from this area of your back as you perform this action. I have advocated that the contractions of both the muscles that are used here be hard. This need only be so until you can use the lower abdominal muscle quite freely. Then you will be able to vary the force of the contraction to meet the relevant challenges to holding the spine in neutral.

One of the main functions of the abdominal muscles is to complement the muscles of the spine and aid in the stabilisation of the spine when we are moving, and one of the major objectives of the Pilates exercises is to encourage them to do this all the time rather than just occasionally, as most of us tend to operate them.

Practice pulling your navel to your spine in this position. It is the very best preparation for engaging 'the core' when you perform the exercises. Pulling the navel to the spine does not mean holding your breath and 'sucking in' your stomach as you may have done as a child to show off your ribs. Rather it means imagining, for example, that there is a strong piece of elastic attaching the spine to the navel and holding them together. However much this piece of elastic is stretched, it still keeps tension in the abdominal muscles.

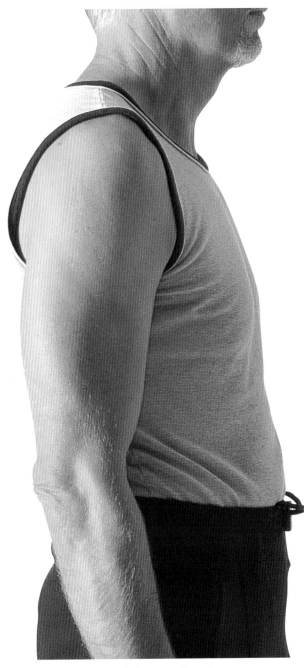

Your abdomen relaxed…

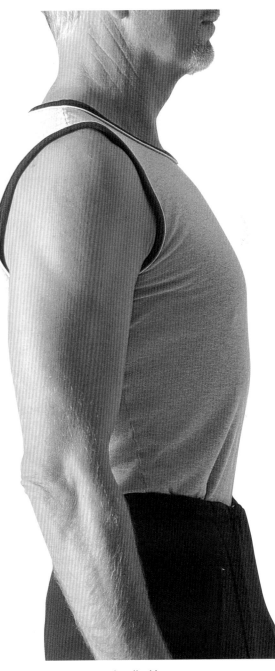

…and pulled in.

Preparation

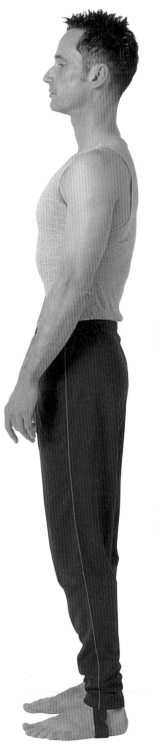

Another useful procedure as you are preparing for the exercise routine is to practice balance. It may seem strange to suggest this as preparation for an exercise routine that is largely confined to lying on the floor and it is not a strictly necessary requirement. It does, however, ensure that all of your muscles and senses are prepared for use. It also begins to re-educate the nerve pathways that control the way we use our muscles so that they respond much more quickly and accurately when we require them to work for us.

STEP 1

Start by standing in bare feet on a hard surface.

STEP 2

Raise one foot about 15cm (6in) from the floor by lifting your knee. Focus on your knee and not your foot, this makes it easier. Make sure you hold your tummy tight while you do this – again this makes it much simpler.

Change legs three or four times. As you get more confidence try closing your eyes – make sure you have something to hold on to as this can be surprisingly difficult to start with.

The other thing worth practising before you begin the exercise programme proper, is breathing.

We talked about the breathing technique in an earlier section, but it is worth repeating in order to get it absolutely correct, as this is the aspect of Pilates that causes the biggest problem for most beginners.

Because when we begin to exercise we are being asked to focus and concentrate, there is an inevitable tendency to tense up and to suspend breathing. As anyone who has done any basic biology will remember this is the worst thing that can happen for muscles that are trying to work.

Incidentally, it also has the effect of increasing the acidity of the blood. Such increased acidity has been linked with a number of the harmful effects that are normally associated with what we have come to think of as stress. So what ever happens – breathe. Even if it is not completely accurate according to the book it is a whole lot better than not breathing or holding your breath. Get familiar with the exercise technique first and then focus on getting the breathing correct.

When asked to take a breath consciously most of us do two things. We lift the front of our ribcage towards our chin and at the same time tense our shoulders. (You can see this for yourself if you stand or sit in front of a mirror and take a couple of breaths). This mechanism results largely from our modern lifestyle that sees us spending lots of time seated and lots of time under pressure or feeling anxious. Although very good if you find yourself confronted by a danger from which you need to run away, as it supplies limited quantities of oxygen very quickly to the muscles, it is not an efficient mechanism for everyday activities. Likewise it is fine for sprinting but ineffective and stressful if you are trying to maintain activity over a period longer than ten seconds or so.

The efficient way to breathe (which means getting maximum oxygen in and maximum carbon dioxide out with each breath out) involves use of the diaphragm and the lower part of the chest cavity.

Preparation

STEP 1

Stand in the relaxed posture as shown. Simply place your hands on either side of your lower ribs, above your hips.

As you breathe out, pull your diaphragm up into your chest and feel your lower rib cage contract. If you don't get it right straight away do not worry, just keep trying.

Alternatively some other techniques may help you to feel the movement better.

Bring your arms, bent at the elbow, in front of you, resting against the lower part of your ribs (like folding your arms across your chest). Hold each elbow with the opposite hand. Holding your tummy firm, focus on your lower ribs (underneath your arms) and try to expand this part of the rib cage as you inhale and contract it as you exhale.

If this doesn't work for you, you may find that using a towel wrapped around the ribs and using this as something for the ribs to push against helps you to get it right.

I believe it is worth practising these elements of the technique for at least one

STEP 2

As you breathe in, push your diaphragm down and try to push out your ribs against your fingers. Focus on moving the lower part of your chest and keeping the upper part of your chest relaxed.

week prior to beginning the exercises themselves. As well as ensuring that you have familiarity with the basics it will give you confidence to approach the exercises in the most positive frame of mind. Once it is performed correctly it has the added benefit of being very relaxing and if you practice lying on your mat with your spine in neutral you may well find that you drift off to sleep.

Finally the most important thing to do in preparation (in my view) is to prepare mentally to spend time performing the programme (at the appropriate level for you) at least ten sessions are recommended before you make up your mind whether it is delivering the promised benefits.

What you need to begin

Once you have done all the preparation outlined in the previous chapter and have decided to commence with your programme, what do you need to do to get started? As with any other task this particular step is often the hardest, because this is where the commitment really counts. So making sure that the preparation is as near perfect as it can get will pay off.

1 If you have not already done so, get the endorsement of your general practitioner. You definitely need this if you have any problem with your blood pressure, any heart condition, if you are taking any medication or if you have any joint or muscular condition. If you are pregnant do not start any new exercise programme and if you have taken no exercise for a long time do not start without first talking to your doctor.

2 You need comfortable clothing – comfortable enough to allow you to lie on the floor, roll over and stretch. Gym workout gear is fine if you feel comfortable in it, but a tee shirt or sweat shirt and jog pants work just as well. What is important is not to be distracted or hampered by your clothes. Do not wear shoes. If you have to wear socks try to get the non-slip variety.

3 You will need a mat on which to lie. However thick your carpet, do not be tempted to do without the mat. You will feel uncomfortable. I recommend to my clients a thick and quite dense foam mat, which really protects and supports the spine when you are lying on the floor.

4 Most of us need a support for our head and neck, certainly to start with. A small firm pillow or a folded towel will do the trick for the majority of people. This support enables you to keep your neck comfortably in alignment while lying down.

5 Make sure you have the right amount of space in which to do your programme. By this I mean make sure that there is enough room for you to lay full length and to stretch arms and legs wide; enough space to do the warm up and cool down which are standing exercises.

6 The temperature should be comfortable for you. You will know yourself best. If you tend to feel the cold make sure you err on the side of warm, if on the other hand any exertion makes you feel uncomfortably hot remember this when you are setting the thermostat.

7 Ideally aim for somewhere where nothing else intrudes. Working out in the sitting room is not going to be good for you if you face constant interruptions from the rest of the family or if the television is on constantly. You will need the right atmosphere in which to be able to focus and concentrate.

8 You need enough time to complete your programme and the warm up and cool down comfortably. Again this is about focus. If you try to squeeze your routine in, when you really feel you ought to be doing something else you will be distracted the whole time. You will defeat the object if you are composing your shopping list or planning your weekend instead of thinking about the exercises. In Pilates, quality not quantity is the key. The secret is a mind and a body that are working in unison.

While on the subject of quality there is a point here that may be important for those of you who are used to other exercise regimes. When you perform the Pilates exercises as described here in the book you will be very unlikely to experience any muscle soreness as a result unless you have not been using exactly the right technique. Muscle soreness can be generated from a number of causes, from excess lactic acid in the muscle, from minute tearing of the muscular tissue or from poor stretching of the muscles. When such soreness occurs it is a sign of inefficient exercise behaviour since the body's energy and resources will now be required to perform the necessary repairs to ensure proper functioning of the muscles in future. Pilates exercises do not generate impact nor do they require the muscles to be stressed excessively. Being asked to increase the difficulty of a procedure by single, small steps at a time challenges muscles. In this way neither muscles nor joints should ever be asked to do more than behave at maximum efficiency so that no tissue damage of any kind should occur.

9 If you have specific aches and pains or particular injuries make sure that you do your recommended remedial exercises before you start on the main programme.

What you need to begin

WARMING UP

A warm up is a very necessary part of any exercise programme. Firstly it prepares the muscles and joints to move through bigger ranges than usual. It also increases the blood circulation to the relevant organs especially the heart. Warm up exercises prepare the heart to pump increased quantities of oxygen, which carries blood back to the muscles and joints, which in turn enables them to perform the extra work that we are about to require of them.

Although Pilates does not appear to be a strenuous there is a temptation to think that the need for a warm-up routine is reduced. Do not fall into this trap. The control and focus required in Pilates can make us less aware of strain on muscles and joints when they are cold and this (in extreme cases) can lead to injury.

Since the Pilates routine uses all of the body parts it is important that any warm up does the same. In order to ensure that I don't forget anything in my own warm up I prefer to start from the floor up, warming the feet and legs through the hips and back and then the shoulders and neck.

Toe flexing

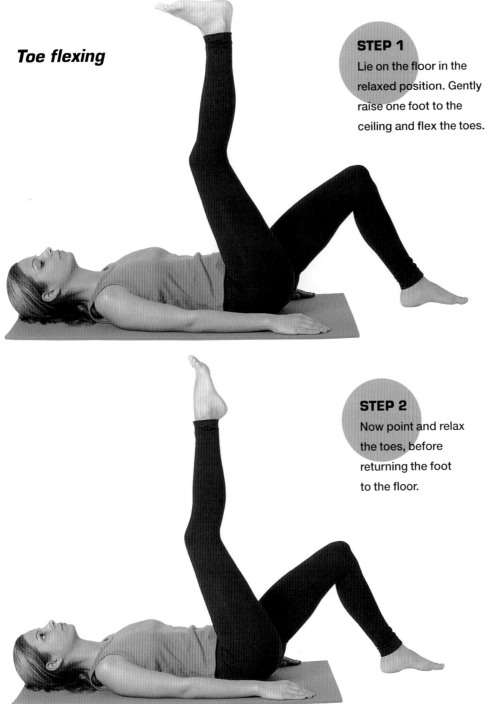

STEP 1

Lie on the floor in the relaxed position. Gently raise one foot to the ceiling and flex the toes.

STEP 2

Now point and relax the toes, before returning the foot to the floor.

Repeat for the other foot.

What you need to begin

Knee rolling

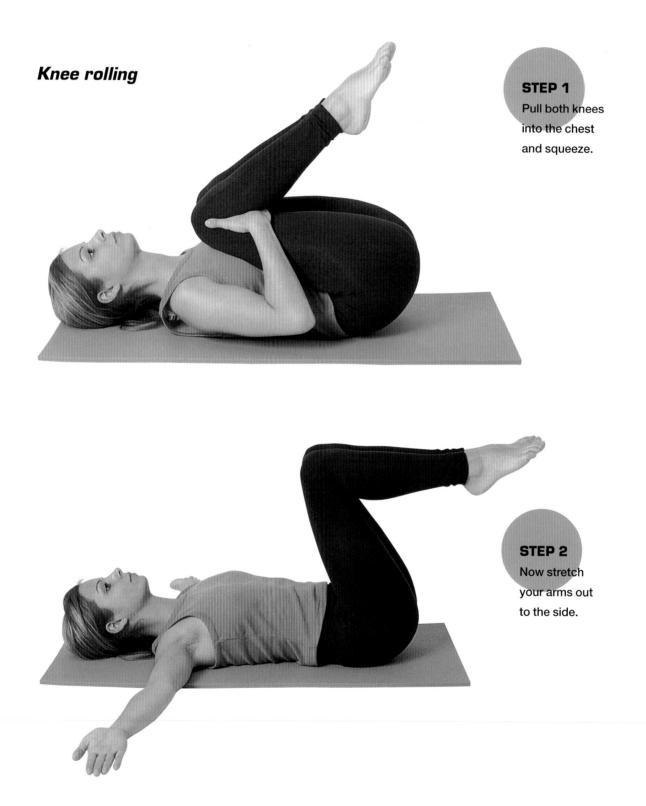

STEP 1
Pull both knees into the chest and squeeze.

STEP 2
Now stretch your arms out to the side.

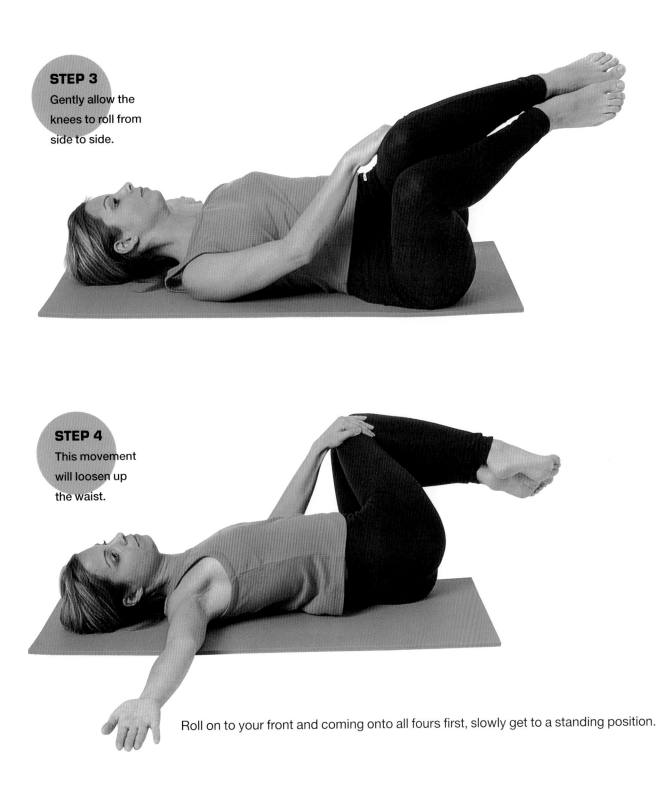

STEP 3

Gently allow the knees to roll from side to side.

STEP 4

This movement will loosen up the waist.

Roll on to your front and coming onto all fours first, slowly get to a standing position.

Ankle rotation

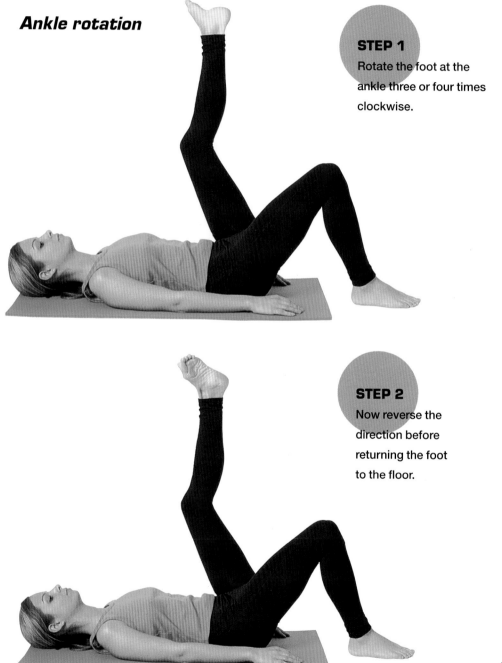

STEP 1

Rotate the foot at the ankle three or four times clockwise.

STEP 2

Now reverse the direction before returning the foot to the floor.

Change feet and repeat.

Shoulder roll

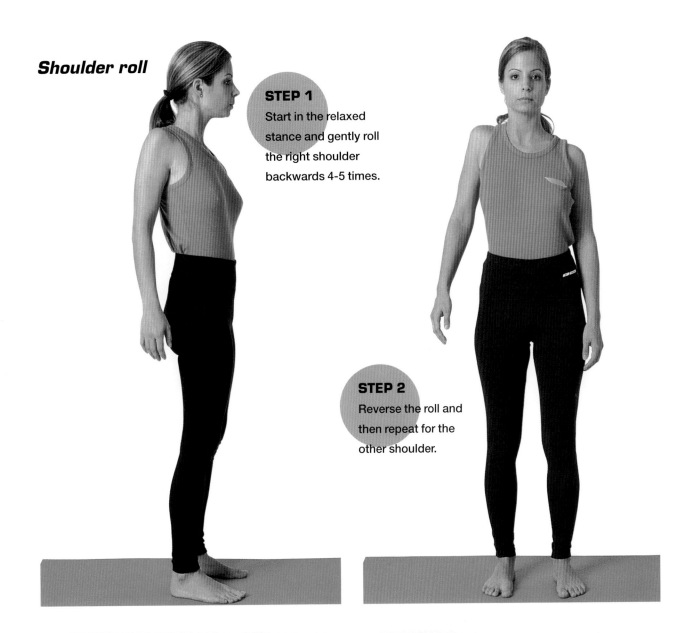

STEP 1

Start in the relaxed stance and gently roll the right shoulder backwards 4-5 times.

STEP 2

Reverse the roll and then repeat for the other shoulder.

Make sure that you use the muscles of the shoulder to perform this exercise and try not to tense the muscles of the neck

What you need to begin

Rolling down

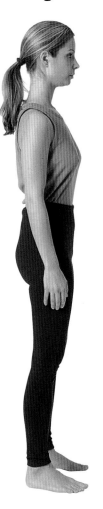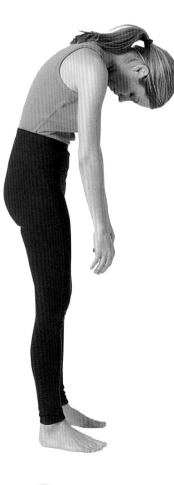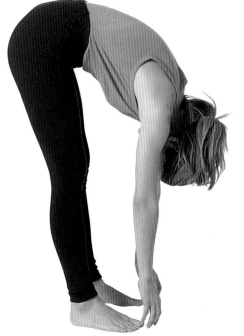

STEP 1
First assume the relaxed stance. Breathe in and pull your navel back towards the spine.

STEP 2
Bend forwards from the hips and allow the arms to hang heavy and pull your torso towards the floor. Breathe out on this movement.

STEP 3
Allow your spine to round as you go down stretching the muscles all along the length of your back.

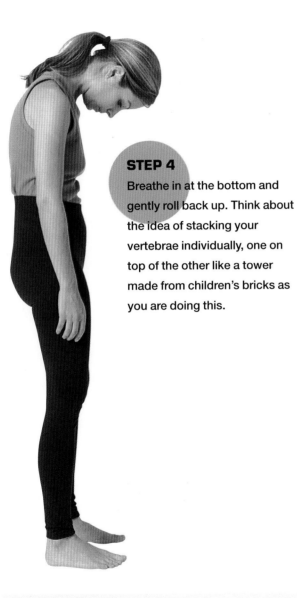

STEP 4

Breathe in at the bottom and gently roll back up. Think about the idea of stacking your vertebrae individually, one on top of the other like a tower made from children's bricks as you are doing this.

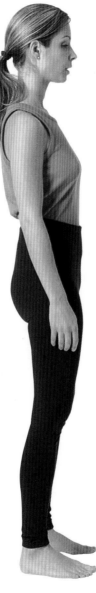

STEP 5

Make your head the last thing to move and as it comes into the vertical position stretch your neck through the crown and up towards the ceiling. Repeat.

If the backs of your legs feel strain, just bend the knees a little until the strain goes. Make sure that you do not push your backside out – it needs to stay in the same place as when you are vertical.

Head rotation

STEP 1

Standing in the relaxed position start with the head facing directly forwards.

STEP 2

Breathe in and gently turn the head to the left, breathing out.

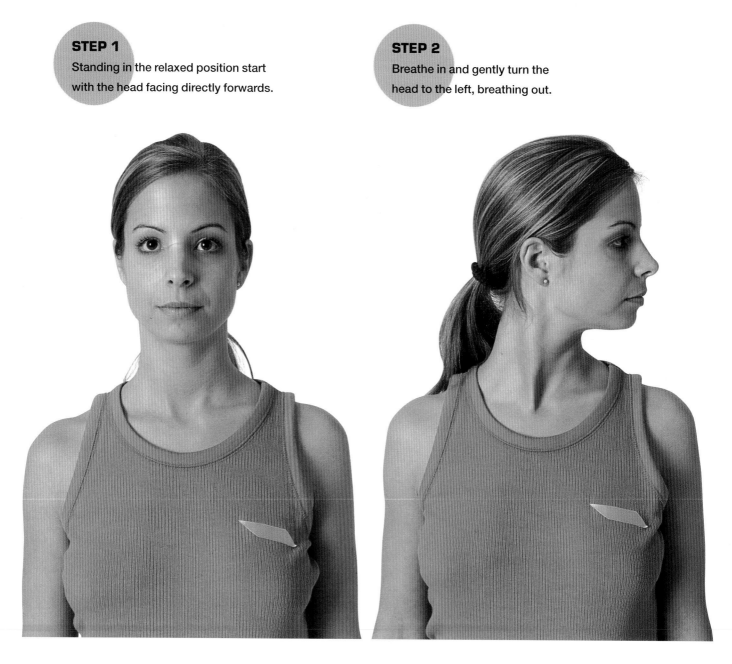

STEP 3

Bring the head back to the centre and breathe in.

STEP 4

Turn the head to the right. Breathe out.

STEP 5

Then bring it back to the centre breathing in. Repeat twice on each side.

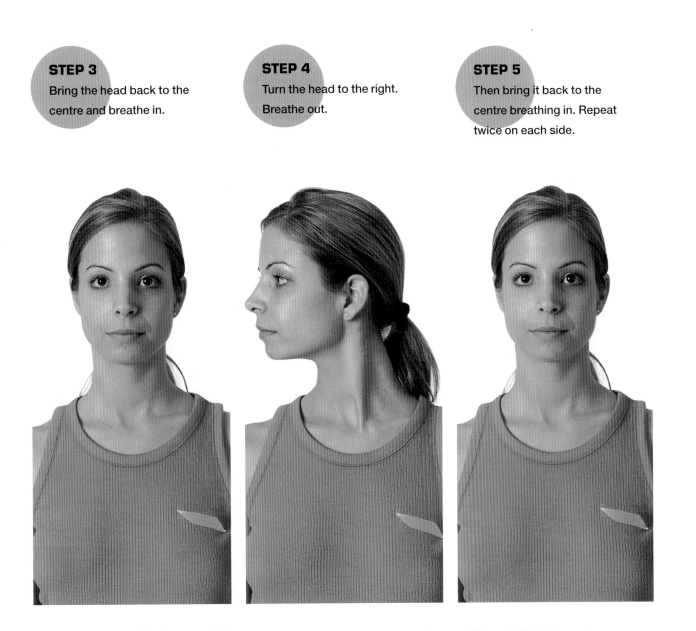

Again keep the muscles of the neck as relaxed as possible and focus on the breathing. This will provide practice, if you need it, for the rhythm of the breathing during exercise.

What you need to begin

Open the chest

STEP 1

Stand in the natural or neutral position as previously. Turn the palms of your hands out so that they face forwards and bring both hands together in front of the body.

STEP 2

Bring one arm to about 11 o'clock, and the other to 5 o'clock so that your shoulders are making a diagonal line across your body. Gently (keeping the back neutral) try to stretch your hands behind you. You should feel a stretch in the front of your shoulders and across your chest.

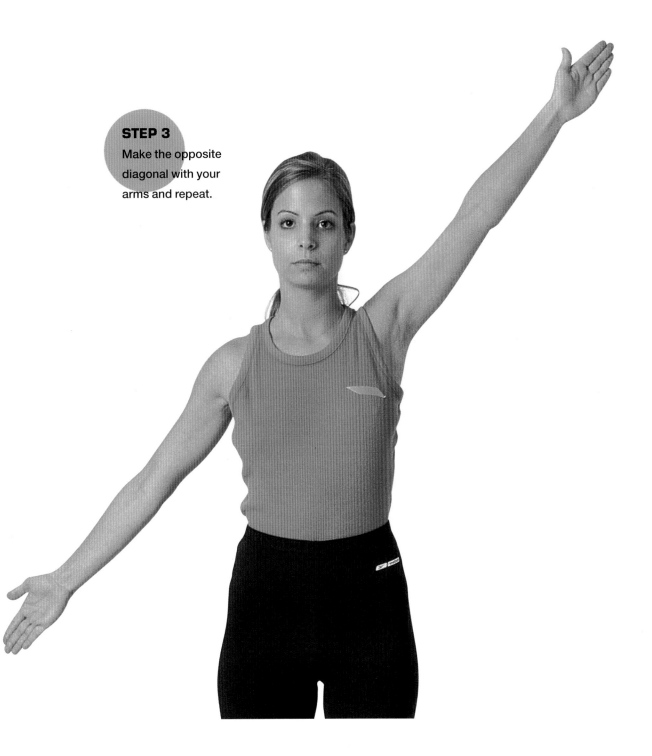

STEP 3
Make the opposite diagonal with your arms and repeat.

The Pilates programme of exercises

Mat exercises for the full Pilates programme number 34 in total and were designed by him to be performed in a certain sequence that he believed had both logic and 'flow'.

For today's unsupervised exerciser (and even the supervised) some of these exercises are far too difficult until 'core' strength has been developed. Where options of a lower intensity are given for any of the exercises always start by trying these first and move on to the full exercise once all the options have been mastered. This allows you to be as sure as you can be that you will not injure yourself. It also ensures that before going for the full exercise you have some idea of how hard it will be and what it will feel like when you do it correctly. If at any stage you feel pain stop the exercise, reread the instructions and retry. If it still hurts – consult your doctor.

It is important for all of the exercises that at the beginning, before you actually start any movement, you are in a neutral position. By this I mean that your spine should be in neutral, your lower abdominal muscles should be engaged, your head should be stretched long on your neck which should in turn be in line with your spine. Your shoulders should be relaxed.

The instructions for individual exercises may not always reiterate this particular point but it is important to both begin and end a sequence re-establishing this posture, in order to avoid the risk of injury that will inevitably accompany any lapse.

The Pilates programme of exercises

The 100

This exercise is concerned with torso strength and breath control. The most important point to remember when you perform this exercise is that your back should always stay in neutral. If you feel pain in your neck or back, go back to a gentler option.

STEP 1
Lie on your back, spine in neutral and as long as you can make it, neck in line. Bend your knees and lift your feet so that your knees come towards your chest. Return spine to neutral.

STEP 2
Lift the head and shoulders from the floor, pull navel to spine and straighten the knees lowering your feet towards the floor to the point where you can no longer maintain neutral spine.

STEP 3
Lift the hands about 5cm (2in) from the floor and stretch them away from the shoulders. Keep the arms straight. Maintain this position for the count of 100, breathing in for the count of 5 and out for the count of 5. You may find that it helps to keep the count if you pulse slightly with your hands.

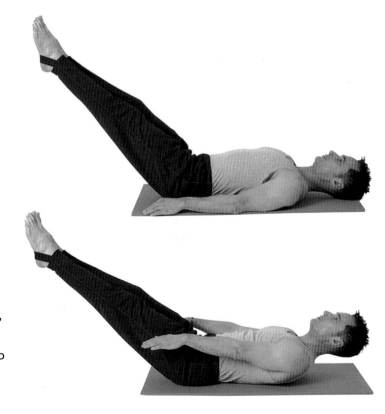

The Pilates programme of exercises

The 100 option

STEP 1

Lie on the mat, spine in neutral, head on the floor. Push your spine in to the floor. Bring the knees towards the chest until they point to the ceiling. Pull navel to spine.

STEP 2

Straighten the arms and stretch the hands away from the shoulders. Lift them if you feel like it and count the 100 as above. If this is too hard leave one foot on the floor, or both feet. Make sure that the spine is neutral. If you find this difficult to maintain then keep the head and shoulders on the floor.

The roll up

This exercise uses the strength of the core to stretch and mobilise your spine.

STEP 1
Lie on the mat at full stretch, hands and arms above your head legs stretched long.

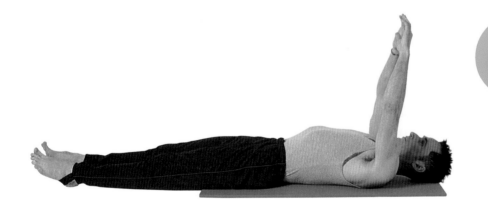

STEP 2
Breathe in, pull navel to spine and bring your arms over your head.

STEP 3
As they point straight to the ceiling, using the core curl your shoulders up off the floor, keeping the movement smooth (think of your spine as a chain being lifted from the floor link by link) and exhale as you come to sitting position.

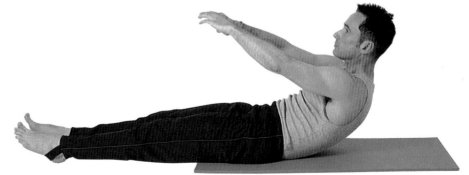

The Pilates programme of exercises

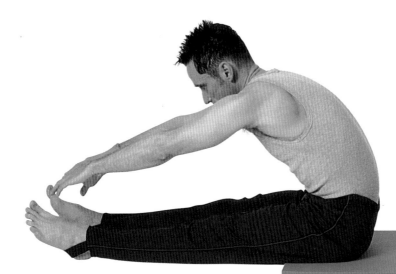

STEP 4

Stretch forwards from the hips reaching with the hands for your toes. Try as you roll forwards towards your toes to lift the weight out of your hips.

STEP 5

Breathe in when your hands have moved their furthest and reverse the movement back to the floor, exhaling on the way down, placing the vertebrae carefully and singly back onto the mat. Try not to make the exercise jerky but move up smoothly and back smoothly. Repeat 5-10 times.

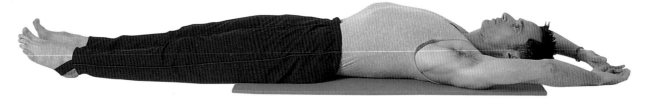

If you find that there is a point at which you 'stick' on the way up then use the option until your back is sufficiently mobile to allow for the movement to be smooth.

The Pilates programme of exercises

The roll up option

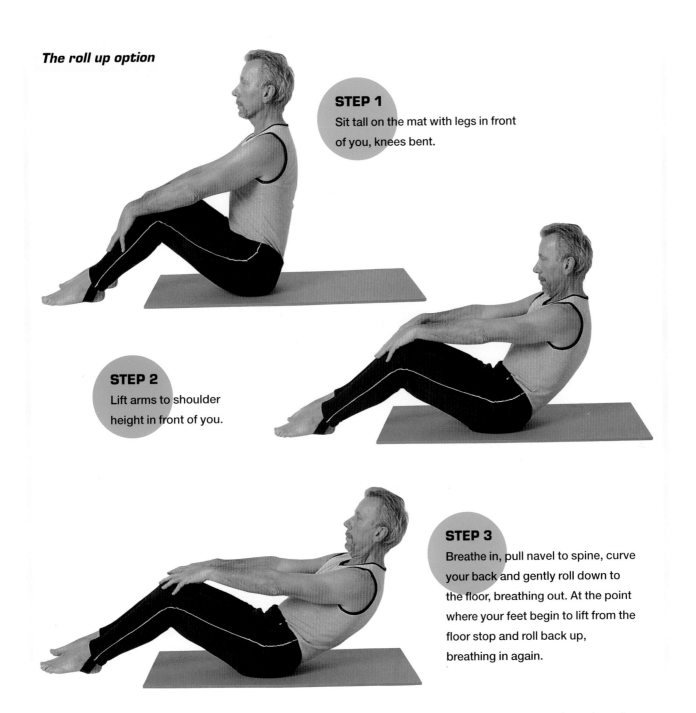

STEP 1

Sit tall on the mat with legs in front of you, knees bent.

STEP 2

Lift arms to shoulder height in front of you.

STEP 3

Breathe in, pull navel to spine, curve your back and gently roll down to the floor, breathing out. At the point where your feet begin to lift from the floor stop and roll back up, breathing in again.

Repeat 12 times in total. Gradually you will be able to curl further back, and then be able to perform the roll up.

The Pilates programme of exercises

The roll over

This exercise also uses the strength of the core to stretch and mobilise the spine. It is, however, very advanced and not to be attempted until you have spent some time developing the core and spine mobility. If you find it a strain you are not yet ready for it.

STEP 1
Lie full stretch on the floor, spine and neck long, legs straight out and arms beside you, distanced a little way from your torso to help support you.

STEP 2
Inhale, pull navel to spine and lift your legs still straight, up past your hips.

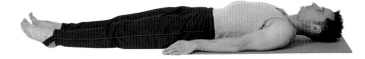

STEP 3
Begin to exhale, bringing your legs over your head until your toes touch the floor. Ensure that you are resting on your arms and shoulders and that you do not use your neck.

STEP 4
Inhale and gently reverse the movement exhaling. When your legs are vertical again open them to about the width of your hands and gently lower to the floor inhaling. Repeat 5-10 times.

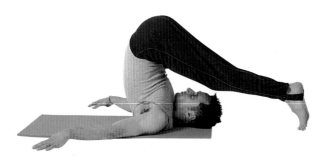

If you find it difficult to get your toes to the floor, simply repeat and you will gradually get there. Do not bend your knees.

The Pilates programme of exercises

The one leg circle

This exercise mobilises your hip joint using core strength to control the movement and keep your hip in position.

STEP 1

Lie full stretch on the mat, arms by your sides, back neutral, neck long, shoulders relaxed. Pull navel to spine. Lift and stretch your left leg to the vertical position, pointing to the ceiling. Keep your navel pulled in. Imagine your leg is a paintbrush and that you are going to use it to paint a circle on the ceiling. Start by making a clockwise circle. Rotate your leg in a very small circle to start – your hips should be absolutely stable and never move. Breathe in for half the circle and out for half the circle. Gradually increase the size of the circle to the point where you can just keep your hips stable. Do 5-10 repetitions then reverse the circle.

STEP 2

Gently lower your leg and then repeat the process with your right leg. Do 5-10 repetitions in each direction on each leg. Keep everything balanced.

The one leg circle option

Should you find that it is too difficult to stabilise your hips in this position, keep the leg that is not circling bent at the knee with your foot on the ground and try bending the circling leg using your knee to make the circle.

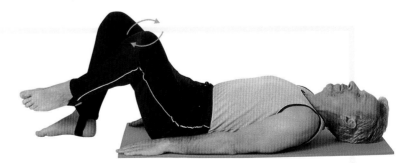

Rolling back

This exercise mobilises your spine and strengthens your abdominal muscles.

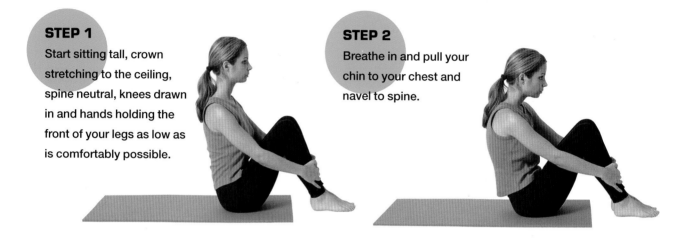

STEP 1
Start sitting tall, crown stretching to the ceiling, spine neutral, knees drawn in and hands holding the front of your legs as low as is comfortably possible.

STEP 2
Breathe in and pull your chin to your chest and navel to spine.

STEP 3
Start to roll back by curling your spine, tilting your pelvis and lifting your feet.

STEP 4
Keeping everything in this position, continue to roll back until your shoulders touch the floor.

STEP 5
Reverse the roll by keeping your abdominal muscles tight and breathe out. Do not move your legs away from your body. As you come back to sitting position make your spine neck and head as long as possible.
5-10 repetitions.

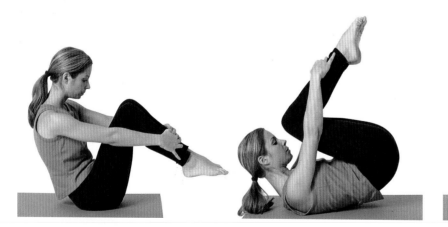

The Pilates programme of exercises

Rolling back option

If you find the above difficult to start with (and most people do) try the following variation to prepare the lower abdominals and the spine.

STEP 1

Start in the same seated position as above, but this time have the arms behind you, hands on the floor facing forwards, elbows slightly bent.

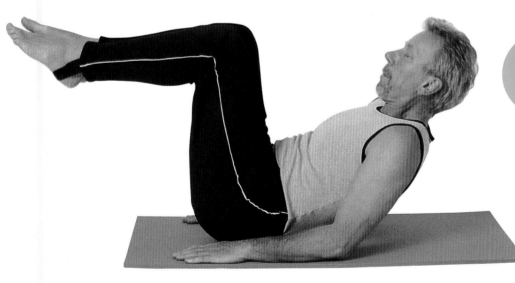

STEP 2

Now breathe in, chin to chest, navel to spine and roll back on to the elbows. Keep the abdominals tight, breathe out and roll back up to seated, pulling the spine long as you come back to the vertical position.

The Pilates programme of exercises

The one leg stretch

The purpose of this exercise is twofold. It uses the weight of your leg to challenge you to hold a neutral spine position. So make sure the focus for you is on neutral spine throughout. This will strengthen the abdominals.

STEP 1
Lie on your back, spine in neutral, knees bent. Think your spine as long as possible. Relax your shoulders.

STEP 2
Pull navel to spine, breathe in and pull one leg in towards your chest holding onto your ankle and your knee.

STEP 3
Stretch the other leg away.

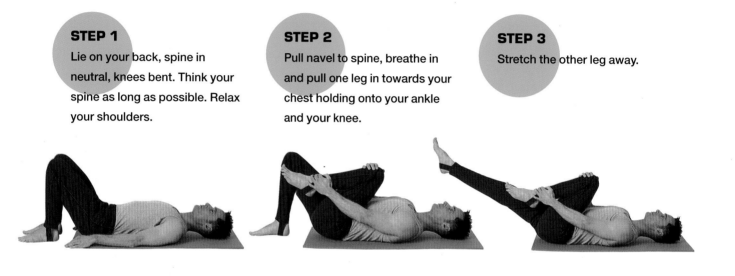

STEP 4
Lift head and shoulders off the mat. Check you are still holding a neutral spine. The more you lower your leg, the harder it is to keep neutral, so raise it if you feel strain in your back.

STEP 5
Then swap legs, slowly breathing as you change position. Make sure you do not strain your neck. Keep your neck and spine aligned. Do 10 repetitions.

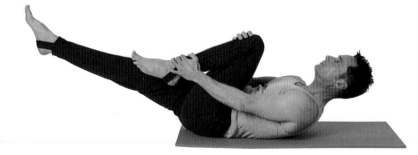

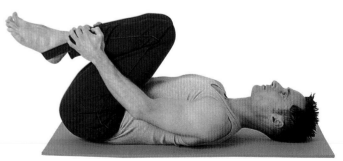

The Pilates programme of exercises

The one leg stretch option

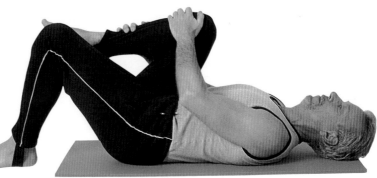

STEP 1

Start lying down, feet on the floor and knees drawn in. Lift one knee and pull it to the chest.

STEP 2

Then lower to the floor and change legs. Breathe as you change.

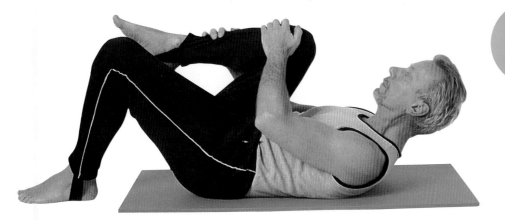

STEP 3

As you feel able, lift the head and shoulders and then gradually move the legs to the position as above remembering that the higher the stretched leg the easier it will be to maintain neutral spine.

The Pilates programme of exercises

The double leg stretch

This exercise is focused on making your back and abdominal muscles stronger, as the movement and position of both arms and legs test your ability to maintain neutral spine.

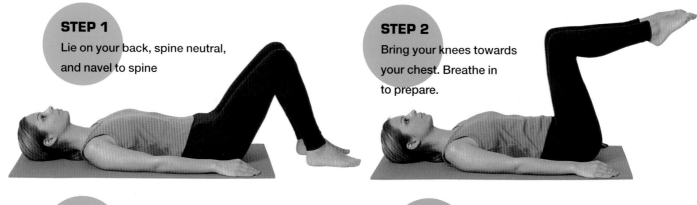

STEP 1
Lie on your back, spine neutral, and navel to spine

STEP 2
Bring your knees towards your chest. Breathe in to prepare.

STEP 3
Now straighten your legs and arms to the same angle (anywhere between 45° and 60° to horizontal) and lift head and shoulders, maintaining your neck in line and shoulders pulled down.

STEP 4
Breathe out slowly and make a large circle with your arms bringing them back to parallel with your legs. Bend your knees and, without pausing, repeat the movement. Do 5-10 repetitions.

The double leg stretch option

For an easier option, keep one foot on the mat (knee bent) and proceed as before.

The Pilates programme of exercises

Spine stretch

This exercise stretches and mobilises your spine. Please note it is not supposed to stretch the hamstrings in the back of your leg, although it will if they are tight, which they are for most of us. If they are tight enough to limit your movement, make sure you bend your knees enough to prevent this and/or sit on a folded towel, which will allow you to perform the movement correctly.

STEP 1

Sit on the mat, feet apart and stretched in front of you. If you can do it comfortably, have the backs of your knees just touching the mat. Pull up through your crown so that you are sitting as long as possible and relax and widen your shoulders.

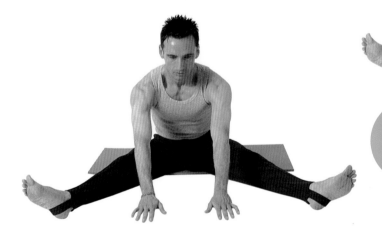

STEP 2

Breathe in to prepare and draw navel to spine, focusing on the abdominal muscles directly below your navel. Lean forwards from your hips. When you are no longer going forwards, breathe in and reverse the movement keeping your spine long and your head high.

STEP 3

Stretch your hands forwards and slowly breathe out as you move. Think about your spine tilting forwards, not bending, so keep it as long as possible during the movement. Make the repetitions flow. Repeat 5-10 times.

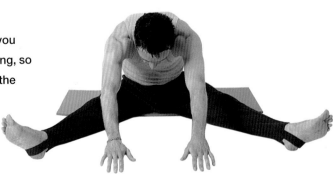

The Pilates programme of exercises

The spine stretch option

STEP 1

If you find that your legs are being stretched rather than your spine then opt for performing the exercise with knees bent and using a towel (or a foam block) as a seat.

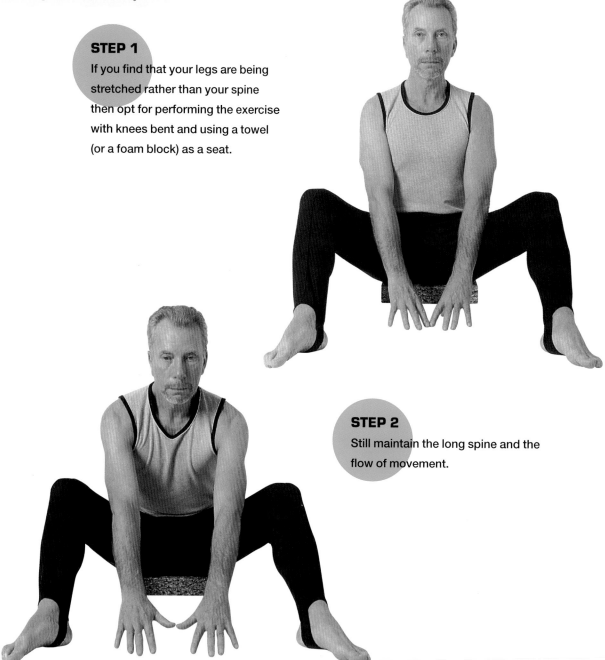

STEP 2

Still maintain the long spine and the flow of movement.

The Pilates programme of exercises

The rocker with open legs

This exercise strengthens the muscles of the core and uses these muscles to produce a movement that mobilises and stretches your spine.

STEP 1
Sit tall on your mat, shoulders relaxed, knees bent, and feet on the floor and about shoulder width apart.

STEP 2
Hold on to your ankles, breathe in and pull navel to spine, lift your feet from the floor and balance on your seat bones.

STEP 3
Extend your legs fully and breathe out.

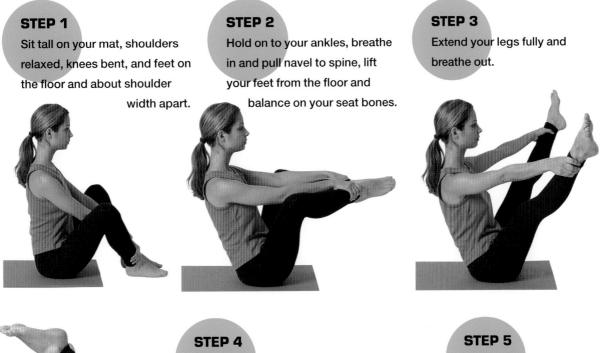

STEP 4
Keeping navel pulled to spine, gently roll back onto your shoulders, breathing in.

STEP 5
Reverse the motion, breathing out as you come back up to the balanced position. Keep the movement flowing. Repeat 5-10 times.

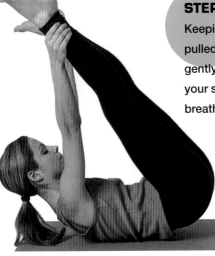

The Pilates programme of exercises

The corkscrew

This exercise uses the strength of the core to maintain balance.

STEP 1

Lie on the mat, spine neutral and gently lift your legs so that they are vertically above your hips. Pull navel to spine and breathe in.

STEP 2

Tilt your legs to one side and make a circle with them on that side, breathing out, maintaining neutral and ensuring that hips stay on the mat and shoulders and neck stay relaxed while you complete the movement.

STEP 3

As your legs get back to the starting position tilt them to the other side and repeat the exercise. Repeat 5 times on each side.

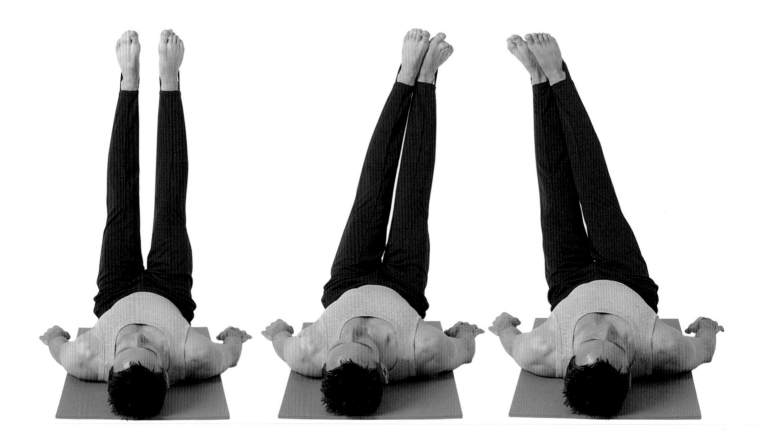

The Pilates programme of exercises

The saw

This exercise stretches and mobilises your upper back.

STEP 1

Sit on your mat, feet comfortably apart and legs stretched out in front of you. Make sure you are sitting tall, crown stretching to the ceiling, your spine as long as you can make it. Open your arms at shoulder height, but not so wide that it stretches the shoulder joint. Breathe in, navel to spine.

STEP 2

Now twist your trunk to one side, breathe out, keep your arms stable in relation to your trunk and keep your hips from moving. Continue to breathe out as you stretch your torso over your leg. Stretch to the point that tests but does not hurt and keep your head low.

STEP 3

Breathe in as you come back to the centre and repeat on the other side.

The Pilates programme of exercises

The swan dive

This difficult exercise uses the strength of the core to strengthen and stretch all the posterior muscles – of your back, your neck and your shoulders.

STEP 1

Lie on your tummy, hands positioned directly beneath your shoulders.

STEP 2

Push in to the mat with both hands and feet. Straighten your arms and breathe in, pull navel to spine. Keep head and neck aligned. Breathe out and lower your chest back to the mat. Use the muscles of your backside and thighs to support your back. Repeat two more times to accustom your back to the movement

STEP 3

As you lift your chest for the fourth time imagine your chest is being pulled to the ceiling. Lift your hands from the floor and stretch the hands forwards, breathe in and then roll forwards onto your lower chest, your legs lift behind you. Breathe out and roll back, lifting the chest and coming down onto the legs. Repeat 5 times.

The Pilates programme of exercises

The swan dive option

STEP 1

It takes some time to get confident and strong enough to perform this exercise correctly, so start with the initial preparation as before and then add in the legs by lying on your tummy and breathing in.

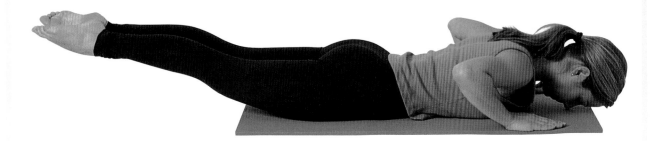

STEP 2

Pull navel to spine then squeeze the muscles of your backside and inner thigh so that your hips are pushed into the floor and your feet and legs (extended) lift off the floor. Breathe out and lower your legs to the mat. Repeat 5 times.

The Pilates programme of exercises

The single leg kick

This exercise is designed to work the large muscle at the back of your legs and the muscles of your upper
arm. It stretches the muscles at the front of your thigh and the abdominal muscles.

STEP 1

Lie on the mat on your tummy. Lift your chest and
support it by placing your elbows on the floor directly
below your shoulders. Press your hips into the mat and
pull navel to spine.

STEP 2

Lengthen your spine, breathe in and kick
the heel towards the buttock. Come back
half way and kick again.

STEP 3

Breathe out and kick your other leg in the
same way. Repeat 5 times on each leg,
keeping navel pulled to spine.

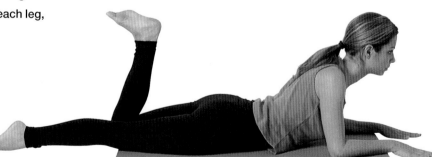

The Pilates programme of exercises

The neck pull

This exercise strengthens the core and stretches your spine. If your back hurts then go back to one of the easier exercises.

STEP 1
Lie at full stretch on your back on the mat, navel to spine and spine in neutral. Imagine your spine to be as long as possible. Clasp your hands behind your neck. Breathe in.

STEP 2
Putting no pressure on your neck, use the core to roll your trunk up towards the ceiling, breathing out.

STEP 3
Keeping your head low, reach forwards towards your toes as far as you are able.

STEP 4
Then, in a single movement, breathe in and roll back down again. Place your vertebrae back on the mat one at a time. Repeat 5-10 times.

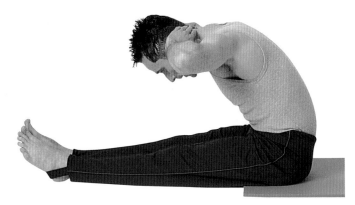

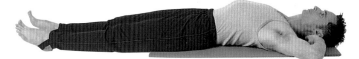

The Pilates programme of exercises

The scissors

This exercise works the core, tests the flexibility of your spine and stretches the muscles of your thigh and also your hip flexors.

STEP 1

Lie on the mat. Breathe out, bring navel to spine as you lift your knees above your hips into a shoulder stand.

STEP 2

Slowly stretch your legs up, bringing your feet vertically above your face – do not let them go past your head.

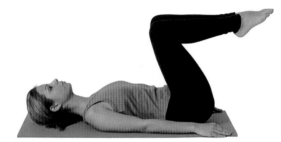

STEP 3

Point your toes to the ceiling. Put your hands behind your hips and make sure you are stable.

STEP 4

Now open your legs, bringing one forwards and one back. Breathe out as you do this and try to move your legs an equal distance – the temptation is to move one much more than the other. Breathe in and change the position of your legs, hips static. The movement should be slow and controlled. Repeat the movement between 5 and 10 times. Keep the breathing in rhythm and make sure you are testing the extent to which you can move the legs.

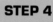

The scissors option

Instead of coming in to a shoulder stand, lift your shoulders from the floor and support your upper body on your elbows and gently raise both legs to an angle of between 30° and 45° to the ground. Go higher if your back feels any stress.

Move one leg down, breathing out. Then change legs, breathing in. Repeat ten times.

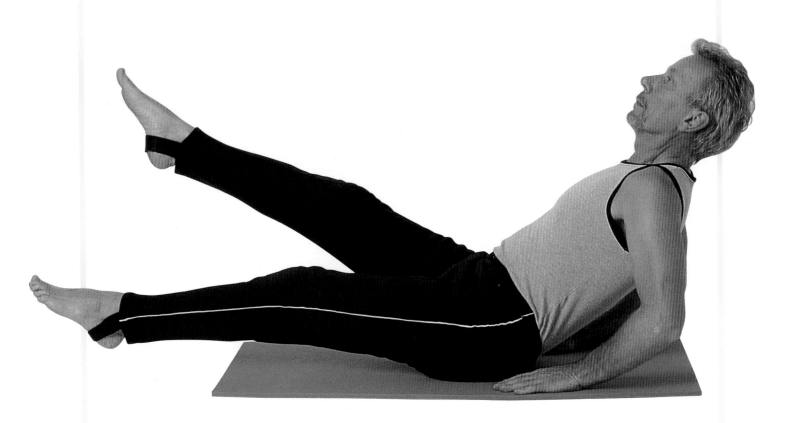

The Pilates programme of exercises

The bicycle

This exercise uses the hamstrings and stretches the muscles in your hip and front of your thigh.

STEP 1

Begin in neutral position.

STEP 2

Move into the shoulder stand position as in the scissors exercise. Bring navel to spine and hold.

STEP 3

Open your legs and then imagine pedalling a bicycle.

STEP 4

Pull the knee and heel of the leg that is behind you in towards your body as the legs swap places. Straighten this leg as you bring it over the top of your head.

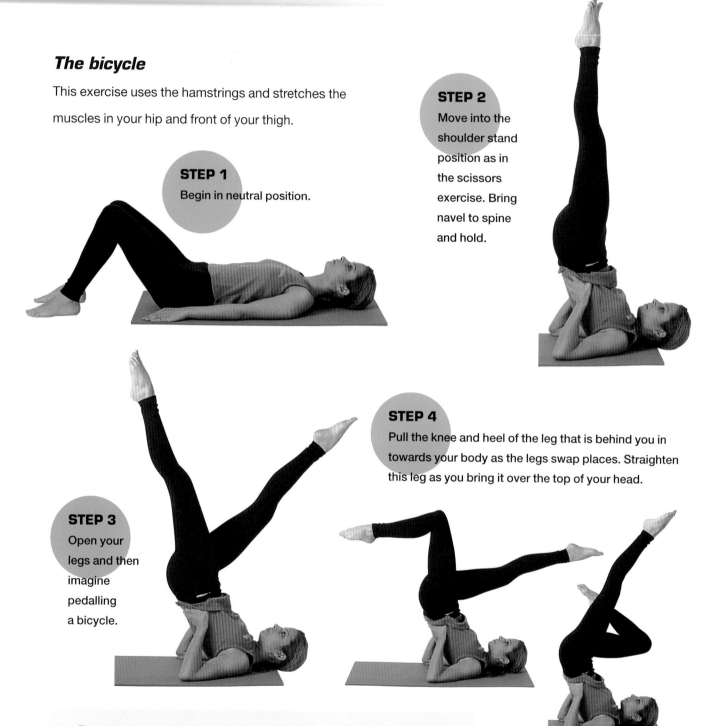

Do not attempt this exercise until you have mastered the scissors

The Pilates programme of exercises

The shoulder bridge

This exercise uses the strength of the core to mobilise the whole length of your spine. The leg movements use the muscles of your thigh.

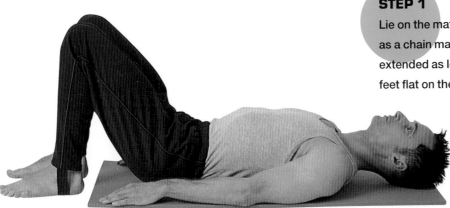

STEP 1

Lie on the mat, spine in neutral. Think of your spine as a chain made up of many links (vertebra) extended as long as possible. Knees should be bent, feet flat on the floor.

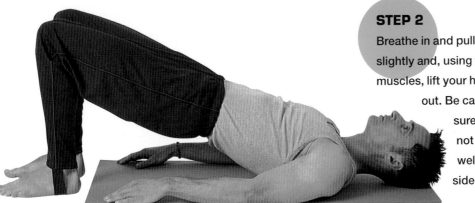

STEP 2

Breathe in and pull navel to spine. Tilt your pelvis slightly and, using the strength of the abdominal muscles, lift your hips towards the ceiling, breathing out. Be careful to lift and not push. Make sure the muscles of your backside are not doing the work. Make sure as well that your hips do not tilt from side to side.

At the top of the movement breathe in. Then very gently and slowly, breathing out, lower your spine back onto the mat one vertebra at a time. Imagine the links of the long chain again being placed one by one on the mat. As soon as your tailbone touches the mat, breathe in and repeat for a total of 10 times.

Once you have mastered this version add on the leg movement.

STEP 3

Proceed as above. When your hips are at the highest point, breathe in, pull navel to spine again and stretch your left leg out level with your other knee. Point your toes. Do not allow your hips to drop.

STEP 4

Then lift this leg towards the ceiling, breathe out and gently lower your leg to your other knee again. Repeat the move 5 times on this leg. Then swap legs and repeat 5 times on the other leg.

The Pilates programme of exercises

The jack knife

This exercise develops the strength of the core. The important thing to remember about this exercise is that it should be performed slowly. It is a prime example of the journey being more important than the destination.

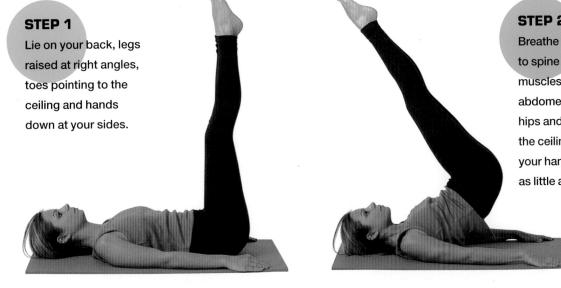

STEP 1
Lie on your back, legs raised at right angles, toes pointing to the ceiling and hands down at your sides.

STEP 2
Breathe in, pull navel to spine and use the muscles of your abdomen to lift your hips and legs up to the ceiling. Try to use your hands and arms as little as possible.

STEP 3
Try also to keep your feet no further back than your head as you are lifting. Do not roll onto your neck but keep the weight on your shoulders

STEP 4
Breathe out, and gently lower your back to the floor. Repeat 10 times.

The Pilates programme of exercises

The sidekick

This exercise is designed to stretch the back of your legs and to challenge the ability of the core to keep you stable and balanced while you move your legs.

STEP 1

Lie on your side. Rest on your elbow and have both hands holding your head. Everything should be aligned – head, neck, spine and legs. Hips should be one on top of the other. Pull navel to spine and breathe in.

STEP 2

Stretch your legs and your head away from the centre. Raise your top leg to hip height and bring it forwards at full stretch to the point at which either your balance fails or the stretch resists the move. The importance of this move is to keep control. Repeat 10 times on each side.

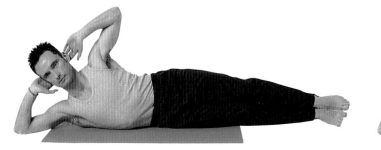

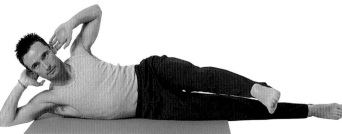

The sidekick option

STEP 2

Perform the exercise as before.

STEP 1

Lying on your lower arm and placing your other hand in front of your abdomen as a support can reduce the stress of the balance.

The teaser preparation

This exercise is all about core strength, balance and control. There is a preparation exercise, and you should be quite certain that you can perform this with no strain before you go onto the full version.

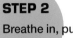

STEP 2

Breathe in, pull navel to spine and straighten your left leg so that it is parallel to your right thigh.

STEP 1

Lie on your back on the mat, spine neutral, feet flat on the floor.

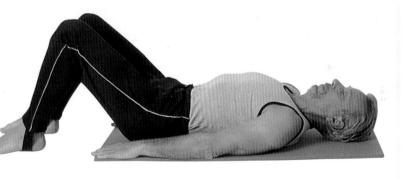
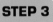

STEP 3

Point the toes of your left foot, reach hands above your head and hold neutral. Breathe out and roll up using the muscles of your abdomen to lift your chest until your torso makes a 90° angle with your raised leg and your arms are parallel to your raised leg. Breathe in as you lower yourself back to the floor. Repeat 10 times, on each leg raise.

The Pilates programme of exercises

The teaser (full)

STEP 1

Once you are confident with this preparation, continue with the full exercise. Start seated, knees bent and spine neutral and as long as you can make it. Pull navel to spine and breathe in.

STEP 2

Lean back on to your seat bones and extend your legs to about a 45° angle to the floor. Breathe out and use your arms a little to help balance you.

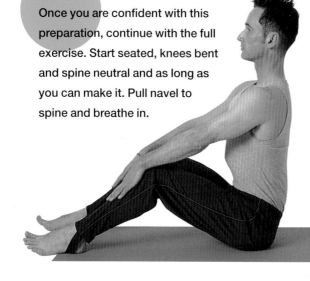

STEP 3

Lift your hands towards your feet until your legs and arms are parallel. Hold balanced at the top.

STEP 4

Breathe in and gently control your torso as you roll it back down to the mat. Repeat, but this time lifting the torso from the lying position. Remember control is the key. Do a total of 10 repetitions.

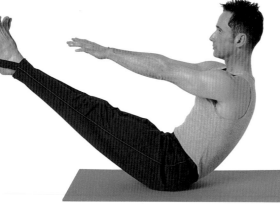

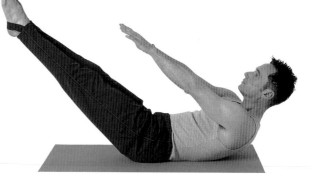

The hip twist

This exercise tests and improves the strength of the core by requiring your torso to remain stationary as your legs are rotated. The position of your arms stretches your shoulders and chest.

STEP 1
Start seated, knees bent, spine neutral and long. Pull navel to spine and breathe in as you move your hands to your sides, elbows slightly bent. Bring your legs up in front of you so that you are in the balanced position. Keep your spine long and stretch your legs.

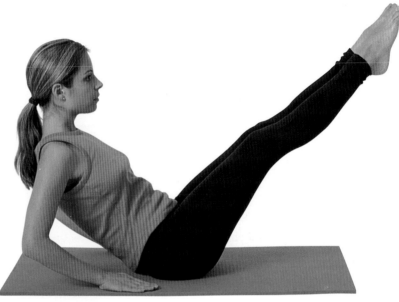

STEP 2
Breathe out and, generating the movement from your navel, start to circle your legs together. Keep the circles small since you want to keep your upper body stationary as you move your legs. Hold the position at the top of the circle. Breathe in and reverse the direction of movement. Repeat 5 in each direction.

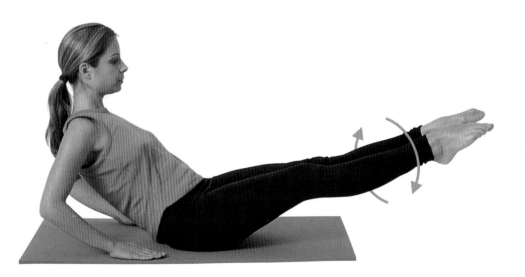

Swimming

This is an exercise for the muscles along the length of your back.

STEP 1

Start by lying on your stomach with your head resting on your hands. Breathe in, pull navel to spine and stretch your left foot away from your hip.

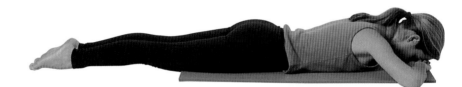

STEP 2

Lift your foot about 5-7cm (2-3in) from the mat. Breathe out and, under control, swap feet. There should be no pressure in your lower back.

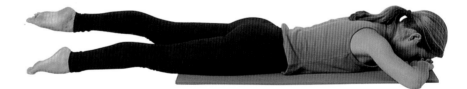

STEP 3

When you are comfortable that you can do this exercise and keep the abdominals tight throughout, introduce your arms. Stretch your arms in front of you and as you stretch your left foot away from you, stretch your right hand, lifting it a similar height from the mat as your foot. Remember to lift your head as well. Keep tension out of your back and make sure that your navel stays pulled into your spine. Do not cheat on this exercise – it is much harder to perform properly than it might appear. Change foot and arm together, breathing out as you lower and breathing in as you lift. Repeat 10 times.

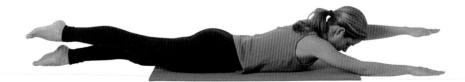

The Pilates programme of exercises

Swimming option

STEP 1

If you find the version above hurts or strains your back then try this option. Start kneeling on the mat with knees directly beneath hips and hands below shoulders. Spine is neutral. Pull navel to spine, breathe in and without moving or tilting your back, gently push your left leg behind you, stretching it to the point at which control of your back and your balance begins to disappear. Do not stretch too far. Breathe out and return to the start position. Breathe in and change legs.

STEP 2

When you can, incorporate the arms as well, keeping your back steady at all times.

The Pilates programme of exercises

The leg pull (down)

This exercise emphasises strength in the core and in your shoulders. It also stretches the muscles in the back of your lower leg, the calf and the tendon in the heel and the Achilles.

STEP 1

Start in the push-up position with weight supported between your hands and your toes, arms extended directly beneath your shoulders. Breathe in, pull navel to spine and ensure that heels, hips and shoulders make a straight line. Do not let your hips sag, nor lift. Do not lock out your elbows. Align your head and neck and keep your shoulders relaxed.

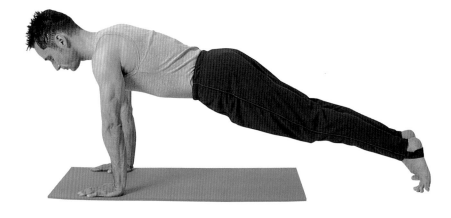

STEP 2

Breathe out, and very slowly lift your right leg. Focus on lifting your heel and on keeping the abdominals tight. This will help you to keep your hips absolutely stationary during this move. Breathe in as you lower your leg and repeat on the other side, lifting your leg slowly and continuously. Your hips should be stationary at all times.

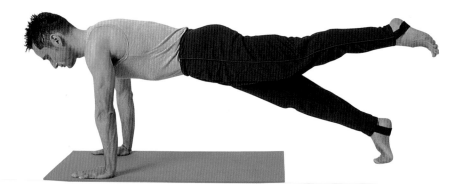

The Pilates programme of exercises

The leg pull (down) option

If you find holding yourself in the push-up position difficult (and most of us do to start with) use the following as an alternative.

STEP 1

Place your knees on the ground and elbows on the floor, directly beneath the shoulders. Breathe in, pull navel to spine and ensure that hips and shoulders make a straight line. Do not let your hips sag. Align your head and neck and keep your shoulders relaxed. Hold the position for a count of 20. Remember to breathe and keep the abdominals tight throughout.

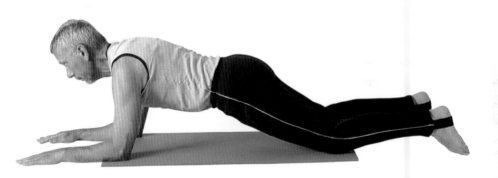

STEP 2

As you gain strength and confidence you can move to a position where the weight is still on your elbows but where the feet, instead of the knees, take the weight at the other end as in the full exercise. From here perform the full exercise, moving the legs but still resting on the elbows and finally move to the press-up position.

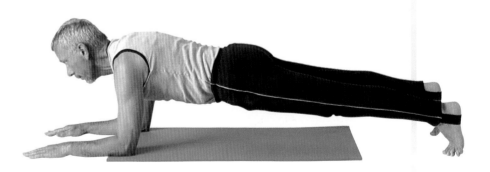

Leg pull (up)

This exercise further strengthens the core as well as using the muscles of your arms and shoulders. It will help stretch your chest and the muscles in the back of your upper leg.

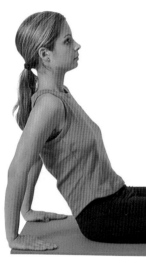

STEP 1

Start by sitting on the mat, legs stretched in front of you. Remember to sit tall and then place your hands about shoulder-width apart on the mat with fingers facing forwards.

STEP 3

Breathe out and lift your right leg to the ceiling. Focus on lifting your heel again as this makes it much easier to use the muscles of your abdomen to achieve the lift. Hold your core absolutely stable with the navel pulled in hard. Breathe in and lower your leg slowly and transfer the lift to your left leg and breathe out. Continue this pattern for 10 repetitions.

STEP 2

Breathe in, pull navel to spine and lift your hips to the ceiling. Ensure that you achieve a straight line with shoulders, hips and heels.

The sidekick kneeling

This exercise tests the ability of the core to hold your torso stable as your leg movement changes your centre of gravity.

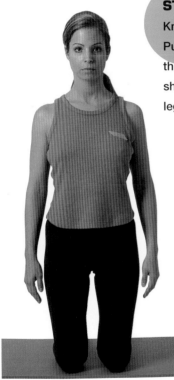

STEP 1

Kneel on the mat with spine neutral and long, knees slightly apart. Pull navel to spine. Lean to one side, moving the hand on this side of you to the floor directly beneath your shoulder. At the same time stretch the opposite leg out to the other side.

STEP 2

Keep your spine long and bend your free arm to bring your hand to your ear. Make sure you are balanced between your supporting knee and arm. Check navel is pulled in to spine and breathe in. Point the toe of your extended leg and lift it to be in line with your hip.

STEP 3

Breathe out and slowly bring your leg forwards at hip height. Nothing moves except your leg. Come only so far forwards as you are able without compromising the position of the core. Then breathe in and bring your leg back. Repeat 5-10 times on this side and then do the same on the other leg.

The Pilates programme of exercises

The side bend

This exercise, like most Pilates exercises, challenges the stability of the core as you move off balance. At the same time it strengthens your arms and shoulders, as they are responsible for supporting the weight.

STEP 1
Start by sitting on one hip with your arm supporting you. Your lower leg is stretched in line with your torso and your upper leg bent with your foot in front of your lower shin one hip on top of the other. Sit with your spine as long as possible. Breathe in to prepare and pull navel to spine.

STEP 2
Breathe out as you lift your body towards the ceiling, pushing down on your front foot and lower arm.

STEP 3
Keep your upper arm extended as you bring it round in an arc until it extends above your head. Breathe in as you slowly lower your body back to the mat. Repeat 10 times and then do the whole routine on the other side.

The side bend option You may find this exercise difficult to start with. If so use the following option.

STEP 1
Start by resting on your elbow and on your knees.

STEP 2
Breathe in to prepare and pull navel to spine. Make sure that one hip is on top of the other. Then press down on your knee and elbow and breathe out as you lift your body towards the ceiling.

STEP 3
Move your upper arm in an arc until it is extended over your head. Move slowly. Then breathe in and reverse the movements. Repeat 10 times and then do the same on the other side.

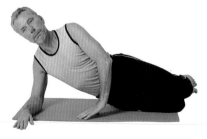

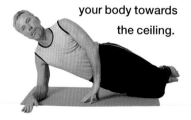

The boomerang

This testing exercise strengthens most of the body's muscles and improves spine flexibility.

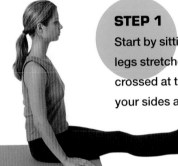

STEP 1

Start by sitting tall on your mat, legs stretched in front of you and crossed at the ankles, arms by your sides and hands on the floor.

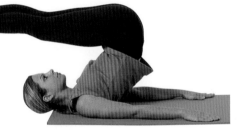

STEP 2

Breathe in to prepare, pull your arms behind you and lean forwards from your hips, breathing out.

STEP 3

Breathe in as you roll back onto your shoulders with feet over your head.

STEP 4

Breathe out and bring yourself back up tall, arms stretched in front of you.

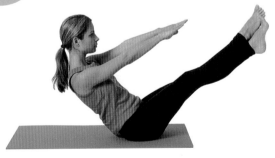

STEP 5

Continue through the movement, leaning forwards from your hips and reaching for your toes with your fingers. Breathe in and recommence the movement. Repeat 10 times.

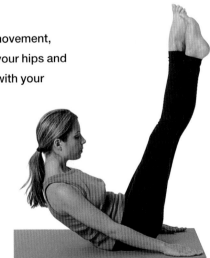

If you find this movement difficult, or if your back hurts you while trying to perform it, stop and go back to one of the other rolling exercises.

The Pilates programme of exercises

The seal

This exercise is designed to increase mobility of your spine and to test the strength of the core.

STEP 1

Start seated tall on your mat, spine and neck as long as possible. Pull navel to spine and move into a balanced position with knees bent, feet in front of you and lifted off the floor, hands holding shins.

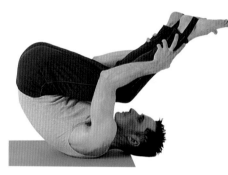

STEP 2

Breathe in and roll back, keeping your body tight like a ball, onto your shoulders.

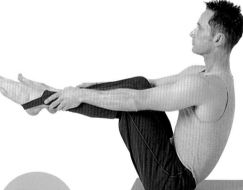

STEP 4

Breathe in, make your spine and neck as long as possible again then 'clap' your feet together 3 times. This makes you hold the balance and focus on the strength of the core. Repeat 10 times.

STEP 3

Breathe out, reverse the movement up and finish in the balanced position. Use your abdominal muscles to stop you and hold you balanced.

The crab

This exercise is another variation of the rolling exercises. It mobilises the spine and, because balance is more difficult in this position, it presents a greater challenge to the strength of the core.

STEP 1

Start seated tall on your mat, spine and neck as long as possible. Pull navel to spine and move into a balanced position with legs crossed in front of you and lifted off the floor, hands holding ankles.

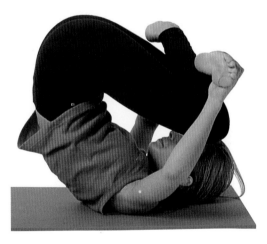

STEP 2

Breathe in and roll back, keeping your body tight like a ball, onto your shoulders.

STEP 3

Breathe out, reverse the movement and finish in the balanced position. Use your abdominal muscles to stop you and hold you balanced. Breathe in, making your spine and neck as long as possible again. Repeat 10 times.

The Pilates programme of exercises

Rocking

This exercise is every bit as hard as it looks. Do not attempt it until you are confident that your core, your back and your flexibility are ready. It stretches the soft tissues of your knees, the front of your upper thigh, your shoulders and arms. It strengthens your back and central core.

STEP 1

Lie on your stomach on the mat. Bend your knees and reach to get hold of your ankles. Pull navel to spine and make sure you hold this throughout.

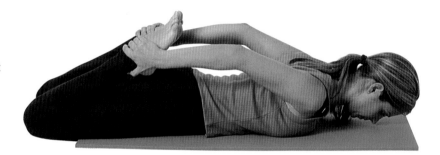

STEP 2

Breathe in and try to reach the back of your head with your feet, lifting your legs and chest off the mat.

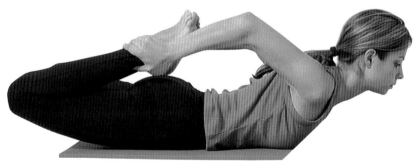

STEP 3

Breathe out and rock onto your chest. Breathe in and rock back onto your legs. Use your ankles to pull you back and up. Rock both ways 10 times. Stretch your back when you have finished.

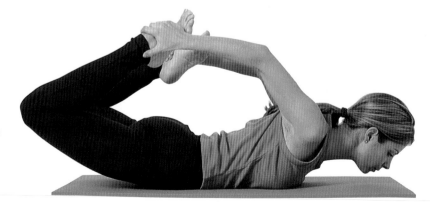

The Pilates programme of exercises

The control balance

This exercise is about stretching and mobilising your back, stretching the backs of your legs and strengthening the core. The key to success here is keeping all the movements controlled.

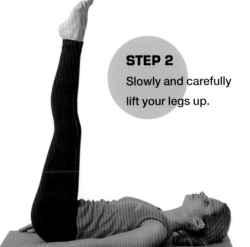

STEP 2

Slowly and carefully lift your legs up.

STEP 1

Start by lying on the floor, arms by your sides, spine neutral and legs long. Pull navel to spine and breathe out.

STEP 3

Bring your legs over your head.

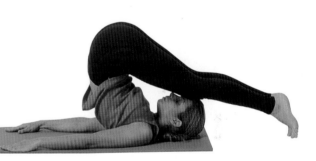

STEP 4

Take hold of your ankles. Breathe in and make your body long, pushing one leg up to the ceiling. Check navel to spine.

STEP 5

Breathe out and change to the other leg. Keep all the movements slow and deliberate. Repeat 10 times. Bring both legs back behind your head. Breathe in, lowering your legs back to the floor.

The Pilates programme of exercises

The push up

This exercise stretches the backs of your legs and your shoulders and, as well as making the core strong, strengthens shoulders, arms, back and chest.

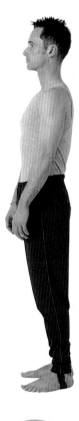

STEP 1

Stand in front of your mat in the relaxed position. Make your spine as long as possible and your knees soft.

STEP 2

Pull navel in to spine, breathe in and roll your head forwards onto your chest.

STEP 3

Continue rolling through your trunk focusing on your spine. Imagine your head and arms are very heavy and they are slowly pulling you down towards the floor. Make sure that you do not push your backside out. If there is stress in your back or in the backs of your legs just bend your knees a little to relieve this.

STEP 4

When your hands touch the floor, walk them away from you. Breathe out. When your hands are under your shoulders and your back is long, lower your chest to the floor, breathing in.

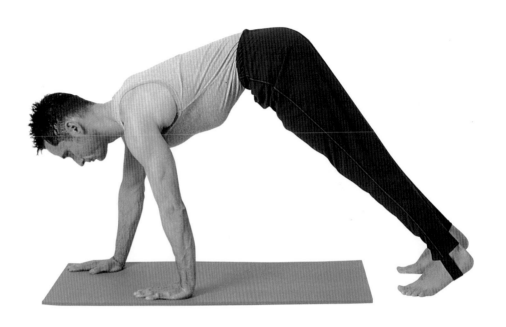

STEP 5

Breathe out and push back up and then reverse the movement, keeping the movement slow and ensuring that your navel is pulled into the spine all the time. Repeat 10 times.

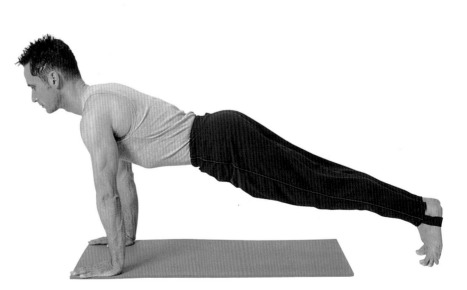

The Pilates programme of exercises

The push up option

For many of us the push up part of this move is too hard so start with the option below.

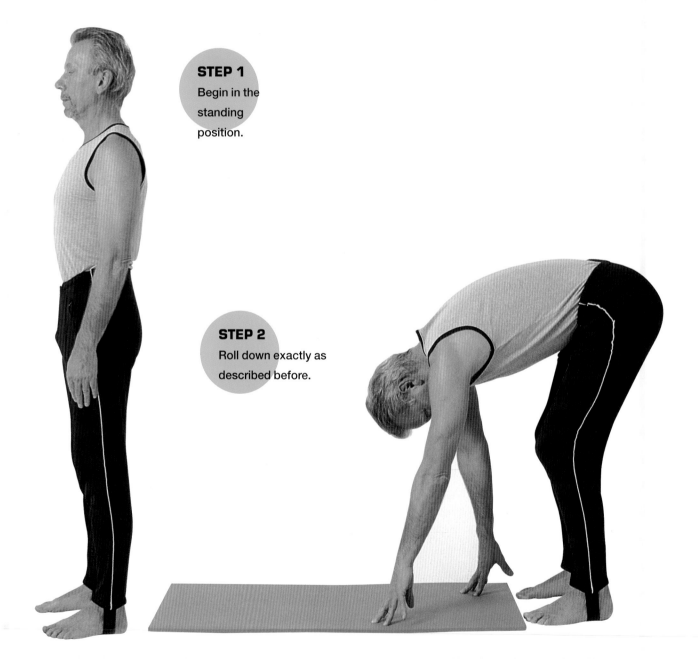

STEP 1
Begin in the standing position.

STEP 2
Roll down exactly as described before.

The Pilates programme of exercises

STEP 3

As you walk your hands across the mat, only go half the distance and come down onto your knees.

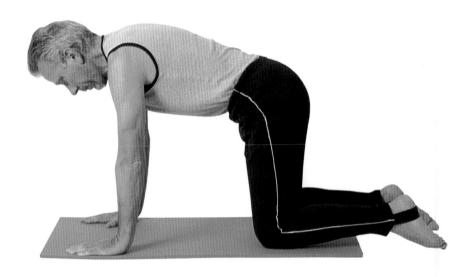

STEP 4

Lower your chest to the floor, breathing in. Breathe out and push up. Then reverse the whole movement as above.

This completes the exercises. Clearly some of them, or some of the options, are suitable for those just beginning, some you need to work up to and some are there to include in your routine once you are practised, strong and confident.

The warm down

The warm down is as much a part of your programme as the warm up and the exercises themselves.

Warming down is important because it stretches some of the muscles you have been using, mobilises joints and begins the process of getting back to the ordinary routine after you have been focused on the exercise programme. Do not leave it out! At the very least make sure that you take two minutes at the end of your programme to simply lie on the mat and breathe properly.

Warm down 1

Whilst you are still lying on the mat repeat the warm up exercises that roll the knees from side to side.

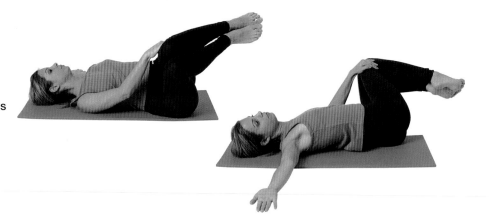

STEP 1
Pull both knees into the chest and squeeze.

STEP 2
Then gently allow the knees to roll from side to side loosening up the waist.

Warm down 2

If you have a ball (as illustrated) and do not have any problems with your neck, stretch out your abdominal muscles. Keep your feet on the floor and curl your back and head over the ball. If this makes you feel faint or breathless at all stop immediately.

Alternatively stretch as long as you can on your mat and hold the position for 20 seconds. Feel the stretch in your abdominals.

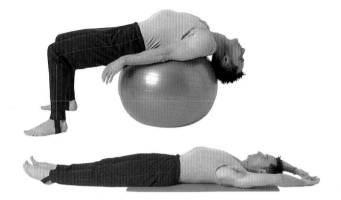

Warm down 3

Slowly and gently get to your feet. Slow and gentle are important because your blood pressure is lower when you lie down and the heart needs time to respond by increasing the pressure again when you come to a vertical position.

Warm down 4

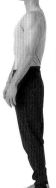

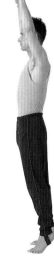

STEP 1
Start by standing neutrally as illustrated in the early chapters, feet parallel, a hip-width apart, navel gently pulled to spine, spine and neck long, shoulders down and relaxed.

STEP 2
Slowly lifting through the spine, raise yourself onto the very tips of your toes and lift your arms back level with your shoulders, breathing in.

STEP 3
Hold for a second or two, then lower arms and heels, breathing out. Repeat 4-5 times.

The warm down

Warm down 5

You can also include the knee lifts from the warm up, if you have time. This is a very good time just to check and try to improve your balance.

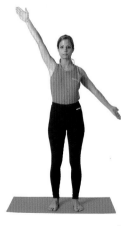

Warm down 6

STEP 1

Stand in the natural or neutral position as previously. Turn the palms of your hands out so that they face forwards and bring both hands together in front of the body.

STEP 2

Bring one arm to about 11 o'clock, and the other to 5 o'clock so that your shoulders make a diagonal line across your body. Gently (keeping the back neutral) try to stretch your hands behind you. You should feel a stretch in the front of your shoulders and across your chest.

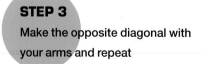

STEP 3

Make the opposite diagonal with your arms and repeat

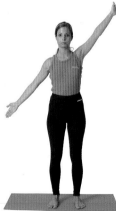

Warm down 7

Start in the relaxed stance and gently
roll the right shoulder backwards
4-5 times. Reverse the roll and
then repeat for the other shoulder.

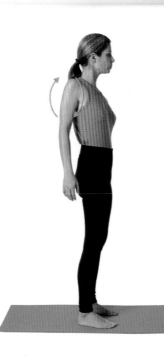

Warm down 8

STEP 1
Standing in the relaxed position,
start with your head facing
directly forwards.

STEP 2
Breathe in and gently turn your
head to the left, breathing out.
Bring your head back to the
centre and breathe in.

STEP 3
Turn your head to the right,
breathe out and then bring it
back to the centre, breathing in.
Repeat twice on each side.

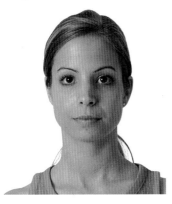
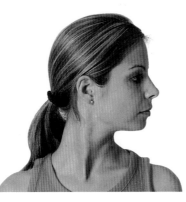
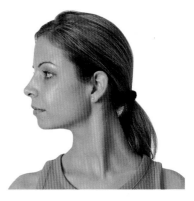

Again keep the muscles of the neck as relaxed as possible and focus on the breathing. This will
provide practice, if you need it, for the rhythm of the breathing during exercise.

The warm down

Warm down 9

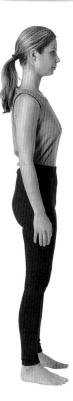

STEP 1

Breathe in and pull your navel back towards your spine. Bend forwards from your hips and allow your arms to hang heavy and pull your torso towards the floor. Breathe out on this movement.

STEP 2

Allow your spine to round as you go down, stretching the muscles all along it.

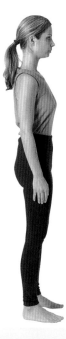

STEP 3

Breathe in at the bottom and gently roll back up.

STEP 4

Make your head the last thing to move and as it comes into the vertical position stretch the neck through the crown and up towards the ceiling. Repeat.

If the backs of your legs feel strain just bend the knees a little until the strain goes. Make sure that you do not push your backside out, it needs to stay in the same place as when you are vertical.

Warm down 10

Finally if you have time, practice some thoracic breathing before you go back to your daily activities.

Stand in the relaxed posture. Simply place your hands on either side of the lower ribs, above the hips.

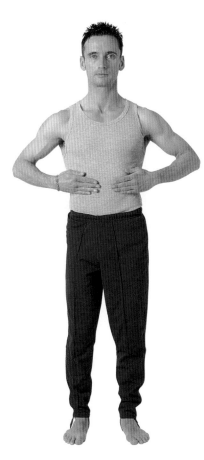 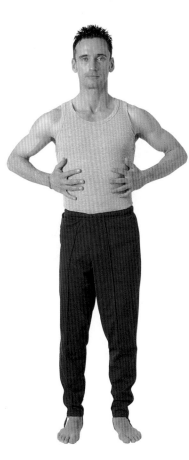

As you breathe in, push your diaphragm down and try to push out your ribs against the fingers. Focus on moving the lower part of the chest and keeping the upper part of the chest relaxed.

As you breathe out pull the diaphragm up into the chest and feel your lower rib cage contract. If you don't get it right straight away do not worry just keep trying.

Deciding on a programme

Regardless of how fit or unfit you are, everyone should start with the same beginner's exercises.

Beginner's exercises

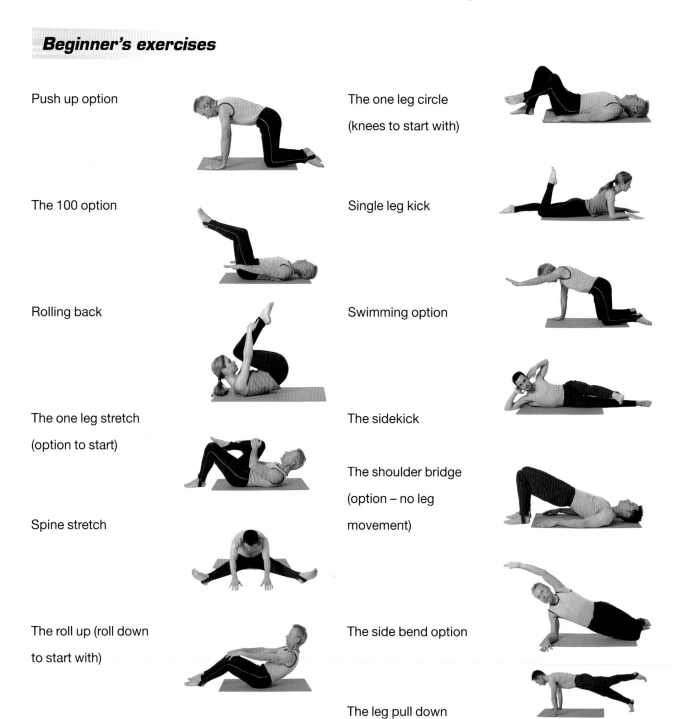

Push up option

The 100 option

Rolling back

The one leg stretch
(option to start)

Spine stretch

The roll up (roll down
to start with)

The one leg circle
(knees to start with)

Single leg kick

Swimming option

The sidekick

The shoulder bridge
(option – no leg
movement)

The side bend option

The leg pull down

Deciding on a programme

Doing the exercises in this order would make a reasonable programme and once you are familiar with the routine the transition from one to the next should be relatively flowing. You might wish to experiment with the order a little making sure that not too many of the 'core' exercises come next to each other and to make the flow better for you.

Intermediate exercises

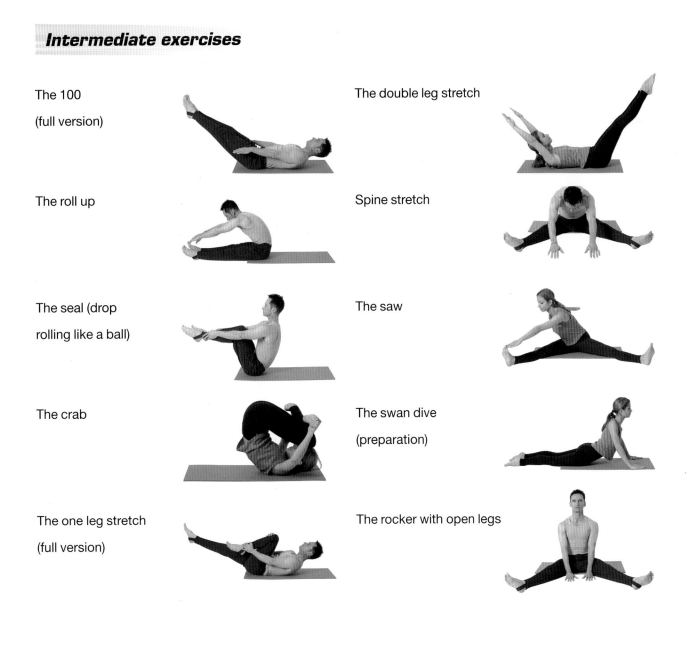

The 100
(full version)

The double leg stretch

The roll up

Spine stretch

The seal (drop
rolling like a ball)

The saw

The crab

The swan dive
(preparation)

The one leg stretch
(full version)

The rocker with open legs

Deciding on a programme

One leg circles (full version)

The side bend (full version)

Swimming (full version)

The leg pull (down)

The sidekick

The leg pull (up)

The scissors option

The teaser (full)

Swimming (full version)

The jack knife

The shoulder bridge (full version)

The hip twist

The sidekick kneeling

Push up (full version)

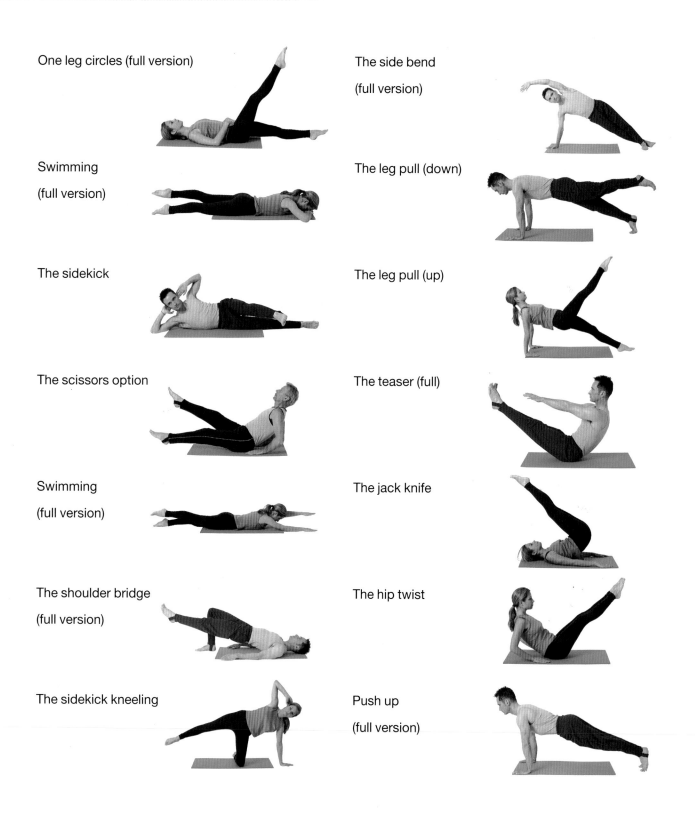

The exercises listed (on the left) are those that have been brought over and/or adapted from the beginner's section.

When you add in, or progress to, the intermediate exercises, the idea is to drop any of the easier versions that you have been doing in favour of the version listed as intermediate. Do not feel that you have to begin all the intermediate exercises together. Add in one or two at a time, as you feel ready. The order suggested above is changed slightly from that used in the beginner section simply to provide a bit more balance. This is not sacrosanct. Change it, if it doesn't suit you, to something that does.

Advanced exercises

Again you can add these exercises, as you feel able. Please do not feel constrained to keep to the order in the list. Nor do you, for any of the programmes, have to include all of the exercises in your workout. You may for example choose to do the total set over three sessions or to practice one or two of the exercises every day while limiting the rest of your workout to exercises specifically for strength one day and for flexibility another. The permutations are entirely up to you.

The 100
(full version)

The one leg circle
(full version)

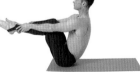

The roll up

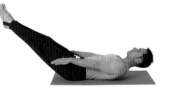

The seal

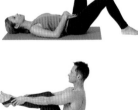

The roll over
Advanced

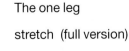

The one leg
stretch (full version)

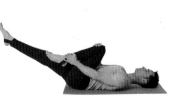

Deciding on a programme

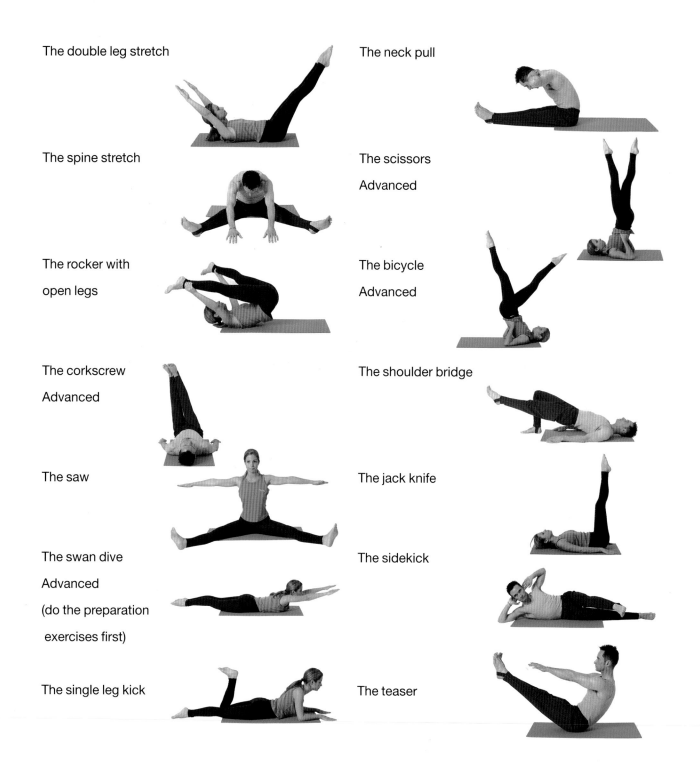

The double leg stretch

The spine stretch

The rocker with
open legs

The corkscrew
Advanced

The saw

The swan dive
Advanced
(do the preparation
 exercises first)

The single leg kick

The neck pull

The scissors
Advanced

The bicycle
Advanced

The shoulder bridge

The jack knife

The sidekick

The teaser

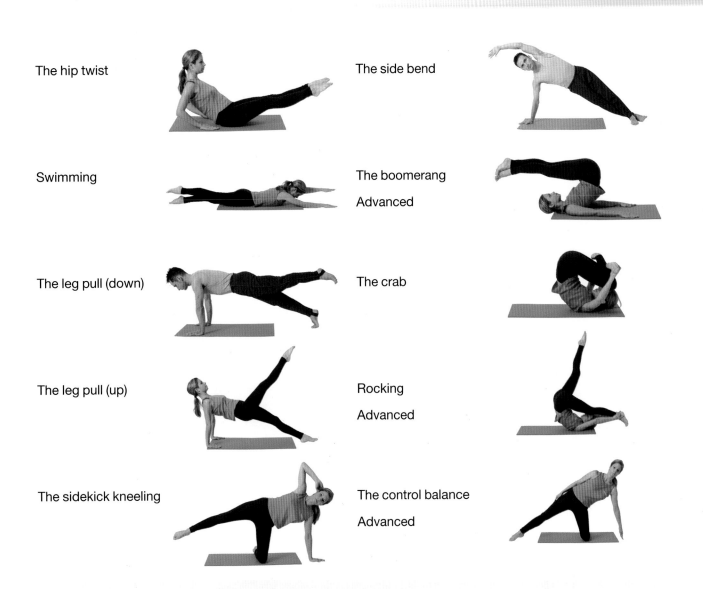

The hip twist

Swimming

The leg pull (down)

The leg pull (up)

The sidekick kneeling

The side bend

The boomerang

Advanced

The crab

Rocking

Advanced

The control balance

Advanced

Do not go on to an advanced exercise until you have mastered any easier version that has been listed elsewhere. If you know that exercises that really use the core hard are difficult for you, then be very confident before you begin advanced exercises that are for the core. Trying to progress too quickly could result in injury and a significant setback in your timetable for achieving your goals. With Pilates, as in all exercise programmes slow and sure approach is the best way to progress. Don't be afraid to move on, but just be careful as you do.

Conclusion

If you have got as far as reading this then I will assume that you have been practicing your programme assiduously and I sincerely hope that you have discovered that the Pilates exercises really do deliver what they promise.

You will have found that you are stronger, leaner, more flexible and that you are looking good and feeling better. The stresses and strains of ordinary everyday life affect you less and you are more in control. With luck your usual aches and pains have lessened. More to the point I hope that you have enjoyed your experiment.

I can honestly say that coming upon the Pilates technique by accident was a great stroke of good fortune for me. It has changed the way I think about exercise myself and has also changed the way that I train my clients to become fitter and stronger.

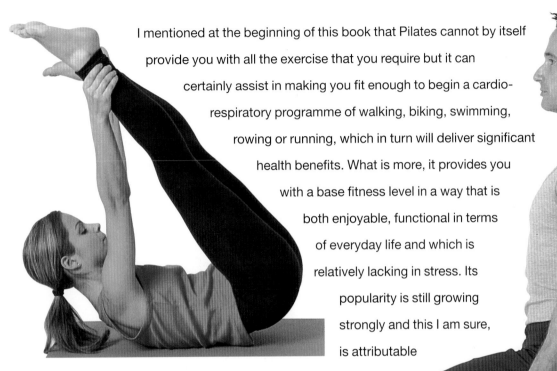

I mentioned at the beginning of this book that Pilates cannot by itself provide you with all the exercise that you require but it can certainly assist in making you fit enough to begin a cardio-respiratory programme of walking, biking, swimming, rowing or running, which in turn will deliver significant health benefits. What is more, it provides you with a base fitness level in a way that is both enjoyable, functional in terms of everyday life and which is relatively lacking in stress. Its popularity is still growing strongly and this I am sure, is attributable not just to fashionable whim, though there is undoubtedly an element of this, but to the fact that it is inexpensive and relatively easy to learn and thoroughly enjoyable.

If you have enjoyed your programme but would like to go further do find a teacher to help you – there are a lot more of us around now.

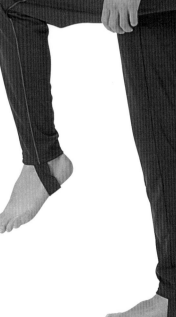

Index

Credits and acknowledgements

I would like to thank Sarah and David for asking me to write this book, and for nannying me through it. I would also like to thank my very long suffering family for putting up with my perpetual bad temper while it was being written, especially my wife Angela who always supports me no matter how much trouble I cause her! Finally I would like to thank my students who have taught me just about everything I know.

The author and publishers would like to thank our hard-working models, Simone George and Mark Slaughter.